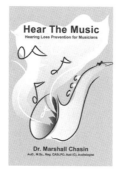

Hear The Music
Hearing Loss Prevention for Musicians

Dr. Marshall Chasin
AuD., M.Sc., Reg. CASLPO, Aud(C),
Audiologist

Director of Auditory Research
Musicians' Clinics of Canada
#340-340 College Street
Toronto, Ontario
Canada M5T 3A9

Adjunct Professor
Department of Linguistics
University of Toronto
Toronto, Ontario, Canada

Associate Professor
School of Communication Sciences & Disorders
University of Western Ontario
London, Ontario, Canada

Adjunct Research Assistant Professor
SUNY – Buffalo
Buffalo, NY, U.S.A.

www.musiciansclinics.com

D0150259

Design: Thong Ling
Project management: Dan Diamond and Associates, Inc.

e-mail: Marshall@Chasin.ca

ISBN 978-1-894801-27-0

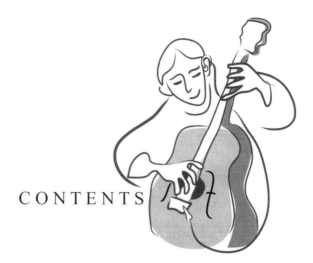

CONTENTS

www.musiciansclinics.com

Preface

"Hear the Music — Hearing loss prevention for musicians" is really three books in one, intended for musicians. The first "book" is comprised of Chapters 1, 2, and 3. It is a detailed explanation of those factors that affect hearing loss, and those strategies that can be used to prevent hearing loss. While the book is written in an easy-to-read, non-technical manner, the information is correct and is well supported by research. The second "book" is in Chapters 4 and 5, and is an accessible summary of those issues and data that are discussed in the first part. Chapter 4 has five summary sheets for various classes of musical instruments and Chapter 5 is written in a "Frequently Asked Question" format. The "third" book is made up of an additional 5 full-pages of more technical information that is optional. The interested reader will gain much from these pages, but skipping them will in no way affect the complete-ness of this book. These 5 pages have a solid line rectangle around the page and are well marked. They are about the decibel, resonances, the occlusion effect, two laws of physics, and more detailed information on in-the-ear monitors.

"Hear the Music" has been written for musicians and rep-resents over 30 years of clinical work with musicians at the Musicians' Clinics of Canada. Hearing loss prevention in musicians is something that has evolved from a fringe, barely acceptable concept, to a central one. Musicians are now, more than ever aware of the importance of protecting their hearing.

Another book of mine called *Hearing Loss in Musicians* (2009), published by Plural Publishing (www.pluralpublish-ing.com) was intended for those who work with musicians.

For those who find this book interesting, but would like more information, I would certainly recommend it.

I would like to thank my family for putting up with me while I was writing. Finally, I would also like to thank Shawn O'Connor who has taught me most of what I know about music, and who tried to teach me the essence of a II, V, I turnaround.

For the interested musician, a website has been developed by the Musicians' Clinics of Canada. The URL is www.musiciansclinics.com. This website was intended for the "high school garage band" but older musicians will find it interesting as well.

I also write a weekly blog about music and hearing loss. It is www.HearingHealthMatters.org/HearTheMusic.

Education about the effects of music exposure on hearing is a cornerstone to any hearing loss prevention program. To support these efforts, the proceeds of this book will go to support educational activities of the Musicians' Clinics of Canada.

Dr. Marshall Chasin, Aud., M.Sc., Reg. CASLPO, Aud(C),
Audiologist
Director of Auditory Research
Musicians' Clinics of Canada
340 College Street, Suite 340
Toronto, Ontario, Canada, M5T 3A9
Marshall@Chasin.ca
www.musiciansclinics.com

January 2014

Chapter 1

Hearing and Hearing Loss

Chapter 1: Hearing and Hearing Loss

The ear is an amazing organ that causes one to suspect that evolution had music and musicians in mind. The ear is made up of "sound enhancers" that boost the treble notes, "sound attenuators" that damp the very low-frequency bass notes, and even special muscles that serve to protect the ear from overly intense sounds. The ear even has a sound "translator" that converts sounds from their normal state in the environment to individual notes, not unlike those on the piano keyboard. In fact the inner ear has individual nerve fibres that are tuned to receive only certain sounds and transfer them up to a part of the brain where the information from these individual sounds are maintained. Figure 1-1 shows the relationship between some notes found on musical clefs and their frequency, given in Hertz (Hz).

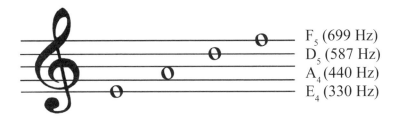

F_5 (699 Hz)
D_5 (587 Hz)
A_4 (440 Hz)
E_4 (330 Hz)

Figure 1-1: Treble clefs with some notes

The jargon of musicians and scientists have long kept them apart. Musicians call musical notes A, B, and C,... Scientists working with sounds call them frequencies. For example, 440 Hz (read as 440 Hertz) is the frequency of the "A" on the second space on the treble clef, 494 Hz for the "B", above it, and 523 Hz for the "C" above that. Middle "C" is 262 Hz and the top note on a piano keyboard is "C" (4186 Hz). They can be used interchangeably and sometimes will be shown as "A (440 Hz)" to represent both the note and the frequency of that note. One convenient advantage of the numerical method is that the number doubles for each octave. That is, an octave above A (440 Hz) is A (880 Hz), and an octave below A (440 Hz) is A (220 Hz).

Another bit of jargon that has prevented communication is the decibel. Musicians talk about "forte", and "piano". Scientists may talk about 90 decibels (written as 90 dB) and 60 dB. Music played at a forte level is certainly loud, but when measured with a special device for measuring the physical vibration in the air (called a sound level meter), it may be 90 dB for one instrument and musician and 110 dB for another. That is, unlike the musical note and its frequency which are synonymous, loudness judged by a musician (eg. forte or piano) corresponds only loosely with the physical vibration in the air—the decibel. It is true that a forte passage has a higher decibel reading than one that is played at a piano level but that is about all that can be said. Table 1-I shows some "ranges" that various musicians may play a forte and a piano passage along with some measurements in decibels. The physical measure of sound vibration is called the intensity (measured in dB), whereas the subjective impression of the intensity of the sound is called loudness. Sound level meters are relatively inexpensive and can be purchased for less than $100. In addition there are many apps that can be downloaded on a smartphone which can do an excellent job. As will be seen in Chapter 3, this subtle difference between loudness and intensity will provide the musician with a few "tricks" to minimize their future hearing loss.

Table 1-I

Loudness Level	dB SPL
ppp	40–50
pp	45–55
p	50–60
mf	55–70
f	70–80
ff	80–90
fff	90–110

What is a decibel?

The decibel is an artificial device that allows us to talk reasonably about the range of intensities that humans can hear. If we merely measure the size of the vibration in the air, the most intense one we can tolerate is about 100,000 times as large as the softest sound that we can hear. The decibel uses logarithms (or logs) to compress this 100,000 range to one of about 100 dB. A measure of intensity such as a dB is crucial because it is the intensity that corresponds to hearing loss and not our subjective impression of it (namely loudness).

The decibel is given by 10 X log (magnitude/reference).

Like the temperature scale (F° or C°), the zero reference is 32 F° or 0 C°. Similarly with decibels, different references can be chosen. For measuring many forms of noise, speech, or music, the Sound Pressure Level (SPL) is used. The reference for this decibel scale is 0.0002 dynes/cm^2. We just need to measure the magnitude of the sound or music with reference to this value. Typically a sound level meter is used which converts vibrations in the air to numbers expressed in decibels. Other reference values are used for other types of decibel measures, and the reference point is usually added to the end of the decibel reading, as 90 dB SPL. In this book, the SPL has been left off for convenience and clarity.

Please see page 6 ☞

☞ *What is a decibel continued*

What is twice (or double) the intensity? Recall that a decibel is 10 log (magnitude/reference). If the magnitude is twice the reference, we have 10 log (2/1) or 10 log 2. For those that like to do calculations, 10 log 2 = 10 X 0.3 = 3 dB. That is, a doubling of intensity is just noticeable as a 3 dB increase.

Humans are rather insensitive creatures and we can barely detect a 3 dB change. Yet, a 3 dB increase means that we have doubled our exposure. Looking at it from a different point of view, a decrease of 3 dB is barely noticeable, yet we have decreased our exposure to the point that we can be exposed for twice as long before damage occurs!

In contrast to intensity, loudness is merely our subjective impression of the intensity, and this varies widely from person to person, and from environment to environment. For example, increasing the bass (or our awareness of bass notes) will significantly increase our perception of the loudness, yet the intensity may only change slightly. In many cases, the musician or sound engineer will turn down to the overall volume (measured in dB) if the bass notes are boosted up. The musician may feel that they are playing louder, but the overall intensity may be less (i.e. at a lower dB). ❧

The Human Ear

The ear is composed of several sections: the outer ear, the middle ear, and the inner ear, as well as the nerves that take sound to the brain (and those that create a feedback loop back from the brain!). A picture is shown in Figure 1-2.

The Outer Ear

The outer ear – the section bounded by the pinna on the outside and the eardrum (or tympanic membrane) on the inside– has two primary functions. They are (i) an amplification of higher frequency energy (the "pinna effect") and (ii) the creation of a resonance in the 3000 Hz region that further amplifies higher frequency energy. That is, the outer ear serves to make the highest octave on the right hand side of the piano keyboard (above 2000 Hz) more intense.

The pinna effect creates a high-frequency boost of sound energy above 2000 Hz. We can exaggerate this phenomenon by cupping our hands behind our ears. There is a definite boost for the higher frequency treble sounds. The physics of this effect are simple and relate to the shorter high-frequency wavelengths reflecting from the pinna back to the opening of the ear canal. The higher frequency sounds not only go in to the ear initially, but are further enhanced by reflecting off the pinna and re-entering the ear. In contrast, the lower frequency energy range, which has longer wavelengths, is not affected by the presence of the pinna and, therefore, is not reflected back to the ear canal entrance. Figure 1-3 shows this net high-frequency boost due to the presence of the pinna, as well as the ear canal resonance. The total effect is also shown.

Structure of a Human Ear

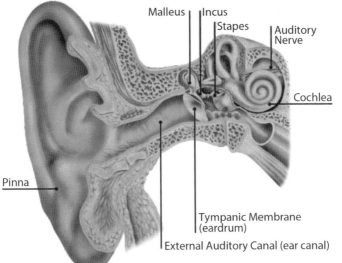

Figure 1-2: The Human Ear is made up of 3 portions: the outer, the middle and the inner ear. Picture courtesy of Bernafon Canada, Ltd.

The 3000 Hz resonance (shown in Figure 1-3) is inversely related to the length of the ear canal (and corresponds to a quarter wavelength resonance, for those who like physics.) This resonance or boost of sound energy is about 15-20 dB.

For people with very long ear canals, this resonance tends to be at a slightly lower frequency than that of "short-eared" individuals. In addition to the ear, almost all musical instruments have these wavelength resonances, that ultimately characterize the sound. That is, a clarinet sounds like a clarinet and not a violin partially because of these resonances. High-frequency fundamental or harmonic energy is enhanced in intensity because of these two properties of the outer ear.

The Middle Ear

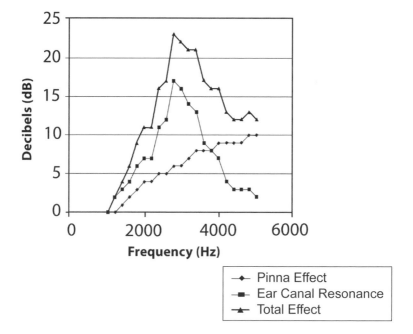

Figure 1-3: The natural amplification of the outer ear, primarily caused by the ear canal resonance and the pinna effect.

Resonance

All tubes and chambers possess resonances, or best frequencies – frequencies that are amplified or enhanced by the container. A pop bottle has a Helmholtz resonance that can be heard when we blow across the top of it. This resonance is caused by the interaction between the characteristics of air in the neck of the bottle and the volume of air beneath it. The ER-series of musician earplugs use such a resonance to re-establish the high-frequency sound, in order to make a flat or uniform attenuator.

In contrast, another type of resonance exists called a quarter wavelength resonator. This only happens when a tube is open at one end and closed at the other. When we say the vowel [a] as in 'father' our vocal tract is "closed" at the vocal chords and "open" at the open end of the mouth. Another example involves our ear canal. It is about 28 mm in length and is "closed" at the ear drum and "open" at the opening of the ear canal on the outside. Some musical instruments such as the clarinet and trumpet function as a quarter wavelength resonator. A clarinet has a "register key" that increases the frequency one and one half octave.

There are also half-wavelength resonators where the tube is either "closed" at both ends or more often "open" at both ends. Many musical instruments, such as the flute and saxophone function as a half wavelength resonator. These are instruments with an "octave" key.

The main characteristic of a wavelength resonator is that the longer it is, the lower will be its resonant frequency. The mouth, when wide open resonates at 500 Hz, and the ear canal (being much shorter) resonates at about 3000 Hz. This means that a 3000 Hz sound, is amplified or made more intense by almost 20 dB by the time it hits the ear drum!

Blocking the tube with your tongue if it is your mouth, or by blocking it with an earplug, will destroy the natural resonance of that tube. French horn players can do this with their hand. This is why all earplugs give more protection in the higher frequencies – the natural ear canal resonance that serves to boost the intensity of the higher frequency sound energy, is lost. The ER-series of earplugs re-establishes this lost energy using a Helmholtz resonator. And, the less expensive, non-custom ETY earplug does this with a quarter wavelength resonator. 🍎

The middle ear has three major characteristics that relate to the acoustics of the sound that a person ultimately receives: impedance matching, temporary reduction of high-intensity sounds, and pressure release.

Impedance matching

Why do we have a middle ear? The primary reason is to match the characteristics of the air in the ear canal to that of the fluid in the inner ear. The middle ear can be thought of as a transformer for a train set. When we play with an electric train set we must be cautious to ensure that the 120 volts coming from the electric socket in the wall is stepped down to match the 10 to 12 volt requirements of the train set. Subsequently, all train sets come with a matching transformer (or simply a transformer) that electronically matches the wall power supply to the needs of the train set. This is known as impedance matching.

Similarly, the middle ear serves to match the mechanical characteristics of sound in the air to that of the fluid in the inner ear. Approximately 99.9% of the energy is lost when sounds go through an air–fluid barrier. This translates to a loss of 30 dB (i.e., $10 \times \log 10^{-3}$, for those who like logarithms and for those who do not like logarithms, it is unfortunately the same thing) and can be noticed when swimming under the water while listening to someone above the surface. If there was no middle ear, our hearing sensitivity would be reduced by about 30 dB. The effects of the middle ear are less beneficial for very low- and very high-frequency sounds.

Temporary reduction of high-intensity sounds

The middle ear also provides for a temporary reduction of high–intensity sounds. This is related to a small muscle that is connected to the stapes bone in the middle ear, called the stapedius muscle. Such a muscle, which contracts with high-intensity sound, serves to lessen the intensity of the person's own voice, especially for the mid- and low-frequency sounds. This is called the stapedial reflex. However, this neurological reflex only lasts for 15 to 20 seconds. Therefore, eliciting this reflex prior to a sound such as a loud noise impulse (by humming) may serve to lessen the damaging effects, but the duration of the effect will not be long lasting. Drummers routinely grunt and hum during playing, and in doing so are eliciting this natural intensity reducer that aids in the protection of their hearing.

There are two important studies (both performed in the laboratories of Dr. Erik Borg in Sweden). One involved studying humans who had a temporary condition called Bell's Palsy. During Bell's Palsy there is a one sided facial weakness and the stapedial reflex is temporarily disconnected. Experiments with these people that create a temporary hearing loss have shown that the ear with the functioning stapedial reflex had much better hearing than the ear with the disconnected reflex. A second experiment involved surgically cutting the middle ear muscle that is involved in this reflex, on one side only in rabbits. The researchers created a permanent hearing loss by subjecting the rabbits to very intense noise. The permanent hearing loss was 30 dB greater on the side with the disconnected stapedial reflex. Possibly the most important factor to explain why some individuals are more susceptible to hearing loss from music or noise exposure than others is because they have stapedial reflexes that are more active and start to operate at a quieter level, thus providing more protection. This most likely is related to a person's genetic make-up.

Pressure Release
A third feature of the middle ear is pressure release. A trapped volume of air such as that found in the middle ear would not be able to respond to changes in environmental air pressure unless a "pressure valve" was utilized. The eustachian tube serves such a function. Typically, this tube is closed and is

surrounded by mucous membrane. When a person yawns or swallows, the tube opens, allowing the air pressure to equalize between the environment and the middle ear. When a person has a cold, swelling occurs in the mucous membrane, thus closing the eustachian tube. Pressure equalization is therefore very difficult during such a time and a temporary mild hearing loss may occur. This problem is more common with children, but adults are not immune.

However, this pressure release can work both ways. Not only can the middle ear pressure be equalized with the environment, but positive middle ear pressure relative to the environment can be established by extreme effort during lifting. Forceful air pressure from the lungs, such as that necessary to lift heavy objects, can cause air to be forced up through the eustachian tube into the middle ear space. This is called the "Valsalva maneuver". Such a pressure differential can cause a slight temporary hearing loss that can actually benefit musicians by acting as a mild earplug. This is frequently noted for wood-wind and brass players who have to continually blow against a reed or mouthpiece.

Problems with the outer or middle ear (such as ear wax build-up, tympanic membrane perforation, middle ear infection, or a stiffening of the middle ear bones) lead to conductive hearing losses. With a few exceptions, conductive hearing losses are medically treatable. Hearing loss related to the inner ear and associated neurological structures is referred to as a senso-rineural hearing loss and, with a very few exceptions, is not medically treatable.

The Inner Ear

The inner ear (or cochlea) is a fluid-filled, snail-shaped structure about the size of the small fingernail. Running the length of the inner ear, over the full two-and one-half spiral turns, is a thin sheet called the basilar membrane. Sitting upon this membrane is the Organ of Corti that contains approximately 15,500 nerve endings or hair cells. The structure of sound transduction in the inner ear is similar to that of a piano keyboard: low-frequency sounds are transduced on one end while the higher frequency sounds are transduced from the other end. Specifically, in the inner ear, high-frequency sounds are transmitted by those hair cells nearer to the stapes (nearest to the middle ear), while those that transmit the lower frequency sounds are found in the innermost turns of this snail-shaped organ. There is approximately a one octave change every 1.25 mm along the basilar membrane (about 30 mm in length in adults) in the inner ear.

One quarter (about 3,500) of the nerve fibers are called inner hair cells and three quarters (about 12,000) are called outer hair cells. Almost all of the inner hair cells take sound up to the brain , and almost all of the outer hair cells receive sound back from the brain. The inner ear presents us with a startling irregularity—the majority of the hair cells are connected to nerve fibres that return from the brain, and only a small minority take sound up to the brain! If anything, one would think that it is the other way around.

Up until the late 1970s, the physiology of these commonly found nerve fibers that return from the brain, was not understood, but more recent research indicates that they function as a feedback loop modulating the function of the inner ear. They alter the inner ear in, as yet not well understood ways that may make the inner ear more or less susceptible to music or noise exposure. As will be seen in Chapter 2, disliking the music slightly increases the potential for music induced hearing loss.

Most people with normal or near normal hearing have emissions emanating from the outer hair cells in the inner ear. These "otoacoustic emissions" can be measured in the outer ear canal (using a very sensitive microphone) and have been used as indicators of hearing function. An interesting finding is that hearing damage from music or noise exposure occurs to the outer hair cells prior to inner hair cell damage. Therefore, an abnormal otoacoustic emission test result may be observed before a measurable hearing loss is detected utilizing conventional pure-tone hearing testing.

It is not clear why outer hair cells are more prone to damage than inner hair cells. One possible reason may be related to the physical location of the hair cells in the inner ear. The inner hair cells sit at the edge of a bony shelf (osseous spiral lamina) so they are not as affected by the motion of the basilar membrane as are the outer hair cells, which sit directly on this moving base. It is possible that this constant movement of fluid and structures of the inner ear eventually causes the outer hair cells to lose their transducing properties before the inner hair cells do.

As discussed above, the inner ear has a complicated neurological structure associated with it that includes feedback loops. In addition to this structure, is the auditory cortex where much of auditory cognition or understanding occurs. It is this central area that is related to an individual's ability to be able to attribute a pitch to a sound. Approximately one person in 1,500 can perform this task with amazing accuracy (called perfect or absolute pitch) and this is thought to be related to the organization of the central structures. People with perfect pitch generally retain this ability despite significant inner ear damage. Recent evidence suggests that this is also the site of many forms of tinnitus (head noises) which will be discussed in more detail later in this chapter.

The Shape of Things to Come

Hearing losses from a wide range of music and noise sources have similar audiometric patterns on a hearing test. The low-frequency sensitivity is either normal or near normal, whereas the hearing sensitivity in the 3000 to 6000 Hz region (near the top note of the piano keyboard) is reduced. Yet, the hearing sensitivity of an individual to an 8000 Hz sound is much better, and like the lower frequencies can be normal or near normal. This "notch" (where hearing sensitivity falls off and then returns to a normal, or near normal level) shown in the audiogram in Figure 1-4, is characteristic of music and noise exposure.

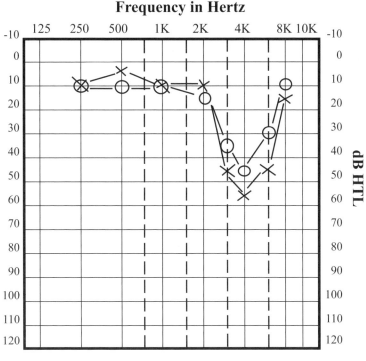

Figure 1-4: Audiogram showing a music or noise-induced hearing loss, ("0" = right ear and "x" = left ear).

Audiometric Notch

Why does music or noise-induced hearing loss cause an audiometric notch? Several explanations have been proposed
for this notch. These include (a) a poor blood supply to the
part of the inner ear that corresponds to the 3000 to 6000 Hz
region; (b) a greater susceptibility for damage of the support-
ing structures of the hair cells in this region; (c) the orientation
of the stapes footplate into the inner ear is such that its primary
force aims toward those hair cells in this region, with the effect
of eventual failure because of the constant hydromechanical
action; and (d) permanent noise exposure has its greatest effect approximately one-half octave above the peak frequency
of the noise spectrum. Since all music (and noise) spectra are
enhanced at 3000 Hz by the outer ear canal resonance, the
greatest loss will be one half octave higher- in the 4000 to
6000 Hz region. Because of these phenomena, hearing losses
due to music and noise exposure are relatively easy to spot.
A bass player and a picollo player may have similar hearing
losses measured on an audiogram, despite these instruments
having different sounds.

A flat "audiogram" at 0 dB—which is a graphic measure of
hearing—would indicate normal hearing. A 30 dB hearing
loss in the hearing at 6000 Hz (an audiometric notch), that is
frequently observed in musicians (and industrial workers),
implies that individual has lost 30 dB of sensitivity for sounds
with energy at 6000 Hz. Such a mild hearing loss however,
would not be readily noticed by a musician. It should only be
thought of as an early warning indicator and not as the end of
one's ability to play music.

Otoacoustic emission testing (measuring changes in the "feedback loop" to our inner ear with very sensitive microphones)
can also be thought of as a very early warning indicator and if
our clinical function is to warn our patients of any impending
damage, then otoacoustic emission testing should be part of
the audiometric battery.

Tinnitus and Hyperacusis

Tinnitus is defined as a perceived acoustic sensation that occurs in the absence of an external sound source. It may be classified as objective or subjective. Objective tinnitus is extremely rare and can actually be audible by another person in the room. This is usually related to a vascular or muscular etiology. In contrast, subjective tinnitus is heard only by the patient. Depending on the study, up to 30% of the population may suffer from tinnitus and 1% of patients report that it significantly interferes with daily living.

Most tinnitus research is designed to develop treatments rather than to determine the etiology, and this is understandable given the wide range of possible causes covered by the one term "tinnitus." Nevertheless, there has been some progress in the development of an animal model by Doctors Pawel Jastreboff and Jonathan Hazell based not only on damage to the outer and inner hair cells, but on certain parts of the brain as well. And for those that like brain anatomy, the dorsal cochlear nucleus in the brainstem may be the generator of tinnitus. Unfortunately for those who do not like brain anatomy, it's still the dorsal cochlear nucleus! Indeed, many researchers now agree that tinnitus is localized in the auditory cortex and that this has been caused by altered input caused by inner ear damage. That is, an inner ear hearing loss restricts the input to the brain and tinnitus is perceived. Appropriate retraining of the brain can therefore reduce the perceived tinnitus. In this approach, a person wears a noise generator that looks like a hearing aid. It serves to mask or just cover the tinnitus. The level of the noise from the noise generator, over a period of months, is gradually reduced, until it is no longer required. Indeed, there are a number of tinnitus clinics that have opened up using techniques based on the work of Jastreboff and Hazell. This is a commonly used therapy, but is not a cure.

The "suffering" of tinnitus is caused by the involvement of the sympathetic part of the auditory system and the limbic system

– the emotional part of the brain. Once the patient becomes emotionally involved, annoyed, or angry at the tinnitus, the louder it becomes. The more annoyed they get, the more they suffer. This has been the source of some treatments – specifically those related to cognitive behaviour therapy.

Some treatments for tinnitus that have appeared in the literature, include intravenous use of lidocaine, various antidepressants, and behavior modification and psychotherapy intervention. The use of hearing aids has been shown to reduce the annoyance of tinnitus in many subjects, as has the use of tinnitus maskers in a lesser number of subjects.

Some people report a strong dislike of sounds – sounds that you or I may not consider to be that loud. In some cases, the fear of bothersome sounds prevents people from going to shopping malls, or socializing with friends. This is sometimes referred to as "hyperacusis". A hallmark of hyperacusis is that it is not always constant and certain sounds seem to be more bothersome than others. Some people are more bothered by sounds when they are stressed or bothered by something else going on in their lives.

This appears to be similar to how some people are affected by tinnitus. And it is no surprise therefore to find that people suffering from hyperacusis have the problem in the exact same place in the brain as people who are suffering from tinnitus. Many of the therapies and strategies to reduce the bothersome effects of tinnitus are the same as those to reduce the effects of hyperacusis. Many audiology clinics offer both tinnitus and hyperacusis treatment programs.

While the approach of Doctors Jastreboff and Hazell looks quite promising, it should be pointed out that no single approach can be considered a cure. An eclectic approach that includes elements of masking, biofeedback, and psychological counseling, as well as various suppression techniques, may be the optimal clinical approach.

Chapter 2

Factors Affecting Hearing Loss

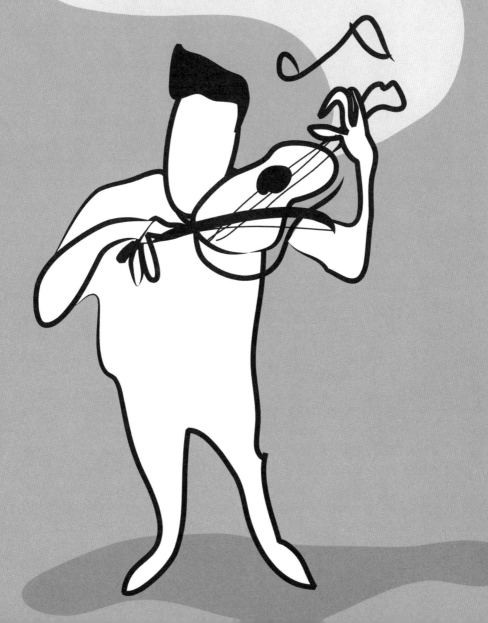

Chapter 2: Factors Affecting Hearing Loss

Introduction

Hearing loss is caused by many different factors. These may include ones that are related to the outer or middle ear, or factors related to the inner ear. By in large, most of the causes that affect the outer or middle ear are temporary and may be medically or surgically corrected. These causes may include ear infections, wax occlusion, or other possibly reoccurring reasons. The two most common causes of inner ear hearing loss are noise/music exposure and hearing loss associated with aging. While being 75 years of age is not preventable, hearing loss associated with loud music or loud noise is certainly preventable.

Hearing loss prevention is therefore a major concern for musicians and for those who work in factories and other noisy places. This chapter will subsequently only deal with the characteristics of music exposure and how it affects the inner ear. Much of what has been learned about hearing loss in the inner ear came from studies about noise exposure and not music, however, most of what is known can be extended to musicians. There are however, some interesting differences between how noise affects workers and how music affects musicians. The differences and similarities will be discussed in detail later in the chapter.

The Intensity Of Music

Clearly not all music is equally intense. Rock and roll is more intense than classical, and both are more intense than jazz or blues. This is generally true, however there is much overlap. The Ring Cycle by Wagner is considered to be one of the most intense classical pieces ever written and indeed, it has been shown that musicians routinely are exposed to almost 200% of their daily dose of noise exposure, in a single performance. In contrast, some rock and roll pieces are rather quiet. In addition, musicians don't just play their own music. They listen to other music and may even have "day jobs" in noisy factories. Frequently professional musicians teach students and that adds to their daily music exposure. And, we must add in their other recreational sources of noise exposure such as hunting, and driving motorcycles. Musicians are subject to a wide range of noise exposure in their daily lives, with music being only one component. Nevertheless, music can have sustained peak levels over 120 dB (in many Rock bands and even during the classical Ring Cycle). Even quiet balletic etudes may have sustained levels of over 100 dB.

The intensity range of orchestras varies depending on the piece of music being played, the performance hall and its acoustical condition, the preferences of the conductor, and the techniques of the individual musicians. Research with various classical orchestras in Scandinavia found that depending on the seating position within the orchestra, musicians achieved their maximum safe weekly dose of exposure after only 10–25 hours of playing.

The intensity ranges in pop and in rock and roll bands tend to be rather uniform since the output is usually controlled by the sound engineer, but sound levels in excess of 120 dB routinely have been measured. With the advent of lower distortion amplifiers, sound engineers are able to increase the volume further without the previous concerns of audible distortion.

Depending on the study, hearing loss has been found in over 52% of the hearing of classical musicians and about 30% of rock and roll musicians. In addition, over 80% of musicians, if tested just after their performance, had a temporary music-induced hearing loss.

Temporary and Permanent Hearing Loss

We all have experienced temporary hearing loss after a noisy rock concert, after mowing the lawn, or even after a noisy social event. A feeling of numbness or dullness in the ears is perceived for a number of hours after the event and there may be an associated tinnitus or ringing in the ears for a period of time. If a person's hearing was to be assessed immediately after such a noisy event, a temporary inner ear (or sensorineural) hearing loss may be found. This would typically resolve in 16–18 hours. Eventually, if a person is repeatedly subjected to intense music or noise, the hearing loss becomes permanent. Permanent hearing loss comes on very gradually and may not be noticed until age 50 or 60. Most people would notice this as a perception that others are "mumbling" more. They may comment that "I can hear you OK; its just that people mumble". Of greater importance for musicians than the gradual onset of hearing loss, is the tinnitus or ringing that is associated with hearing loss, and less commonly, pitch perception problems, where a musician may hear a "C" slightly flat, as if it were a "B".

In the research literature, most of the studies in this subject area relate either to hearing loss in large scale field studies or from experiments with animals. The most common type of experiment is to give an intense noise to create a temporary hearing loss referred to as a temporary threshold shift (TTS). As the name implies, TTS is the temporary elevation of the hearing threshold and can be thought of as an early warning sign for a potentially permanent threshold shift (PTS).

Temporary and permanent inner ear hearing losses typically occur at approximately one half octave above the stimulus peak (most intense) frequency and, as noted in Chapter 1, this would be in the 3000–6000 Hz region for most noise sources and for music. That is, regardless of whether a person was playing the bass or a picollo, the hearing loss would be in the 3000-6000 Hz region—near the top note of the piano keyboard. Above this region, the hearing would return to normal. Therefore a musician with a very significant hearing loss at 4000 Hz, may have excellent hearing at 15,000 Hz or even 20,000 Hz (the upper range of hearing for humans). This is one reason why hearing is not routinely tested at these ultra-high frequencies. There is no diagnostic information up in that rarified region.

The relationship between TTS and PTS is not well defined. A musician or concert goer that has a large temporary hearing loss (e.g., a muffled feeling) after a concert is not necessarily more prone to a future permanent hearing loss than someone else who only experiences a slight temporary hearing loss. However, researchers can say that if music or noise does not cause TTS, then it will also not cause PTS.

If you look at the physiology of what exactly happens in the cochlea with TTS and PTS we see that there are different mechanisms involved. TTS derives from several mechanisms that may included an overabundance of a chemical called glutamate. High levels of glutamate can be toxic to the ear and until the body carries this away, there may be a temporary loss. Permanent hearing loss derives from other mechanisms such as a destruction of hair cells and understandably this would be permanent. So it is not surprising that TTS and PTS would not be highly correlated.

How loud does music have to be in order to be damaging?

This is an area where the subjective impression of the intensity, known as loudness, may mislead us. Recall (from Chapter 1) that it is intensity that is related to hearing loss and not loudness. Whereas intensity is a measure of the physical vibration in the air, loudness is merely our subjective impression of the intensity. A dial tone on a telephone is about 85 dB, and a MP-3 player on volume 3 may be about 85 dB. Clearly 85 dB does not sound loud, but it is intense. In fact, if one would listen to 85 dB for about 40 hours each week, for 1 year, one would expect to have a permanent hearing loss.

Several factors can affect our subjective impression of the intensity of the music. One is the presence of background noise. Imagine yourself in a car going at the speed limit on a highway with the radio set to a comfortable loudness. The car comes to a stop (hopefully not due to an accident) and the radio sounds much louder. In both cases the intensity was the same, but due to the presence of wind and car noise, while driving at the speed limit, our impression was altered. At the speed limit, our most comfortable listening level may be at 90 dB, but when at rest, it may only be at about 75 dB. The important thing to note is that whether the car is moving or not, as long as the intensity is the same, the potential damage is the same, regardless of one's impression of the intensity. And, certain types of music are supposed to be "louder" than other types, so expectation of loudness can be an issue. Table 2-I shows the permanent hearing loss at 4000 Hz for a number of different studies at three exposure levels (85 dB, 90 dB, and 95 dB).

	Passchier-Vermeer	Robinson	Baughn	NIOSH	ISO R-1999
85 dBA	8	6	9	5	6
90 dBA	15	12	14	11	11
95 dBA	23	18	17	20	21

Table 2-I: Prediced permanent hearing loss as a function of three intensity levels (from 85-95 dBA) for five different studies/models of hearing loss.

But,... I don't listen or play my music for 40 hours each week!

There is a relationship between how intense the music or noise is and how long one can be exposed to it. This has been called the exchange rate, since we can figuratively "exchange" a higher intensity level for a shorter time of exposure. Simply stated, the exchange rate says that for every increase in intensity of 3 dB, we should only be exposed one half the time. For example, if we listen to, or play music for 40 hours each week at 85 dB, this is identical to listening to music, for 20 hours each week at 88 dB, 10 hours each week at 91 dB, and 5 hours each week at 94 dB. We may not play or listen to music for 40 hours each week, but even 5 hours each week at 94 dB (about half volume on an MP-3 player) may create a permanent hearing loss. The other way of looking at this, is if we can reduce the sound level by only 3 dB (see Chapter 3 for some strategies) we can be exposed for twice as long before the same damage occurs!

That may be true for factory workers, but I'm a musician. It can't be as bad for music!

Actually, musicians are different from factory workers in several areas which do indeed make them slightly less susceptible to music exposure than their industrial colleagues. Music tends to be intermittent, with loud passages, and quiet passages intermixed. It is this intermittency that causes the music to be slightly less damaging than an equal intensity of noise for a similar length of time. Researchers have calculated how quiet the sound needs to be in order to have no damage (no TTS). These values along with typical intensities of 3 instruments, are shown in Table 2-II. Depending on the musical piece, the orchestra size, and one's exact position in the orchestra pit or stage, there may be some relief from hearing loss by the intermittent nature of music. Certainly musicians in smaller groups such as quartets would receive a greater relief from the intermittent nature of the music than would musicians in a large orchestra or rock band. Those in rock bands may never achieve an effective quiet level.

Whether the full benefit of intermittent noise or music can be achieved by that individual or not, undoubtedly some relief is provided to musicians that is not shared by those people working in a noisy factory. A major reason why intermittent sound, like music, is less damaging than factory noise exposure is related to the function of the stapedial reflex which reduces the music intensity in the middle ear.

A major difference between noise and music exposure is that music is presumably enjoyable. This preference for music is the source of some interesting findings with respect to temporary hearing loss or TTS. In a landmark study, a German researcher named Hörmann studied the emotional effects on

Frequency (Hz)	Effective Quiet (dBA)	Clarinet (dBA)	Violin (dBA)	Trumpet (dBA)
250	77	72–82	75–84	75–98
500	75–85	73–84	75–87	76–98
1k	81–82	69–81	71–78	70–87
2k	77–78	66–74	70–74	66–77
4k	74–76	56–62	59–65	60–67

Table 2-II: Estimates of "Effective Quiet" – a level that would cause no hearing loss – and the range of intensities of three musical instruments. (see text for explanation).

TTS at 4000 Hz. One group of subjects was given a 95 dB noise for 30 minutes as a "reward" for performing a task and another group was given the same noise as a "punishment." The TTS for the punishment group was 18.1 dB but that for the reward group was only 12.8 dB. That is, the "noise" exposure was the same but one group viewed it positively and the other, negatively. The group that viewed it negatively had a greater temporary hearing loss! This type of study has been performed many times over the years with noise and music of equal energy, and with comparing groups of subjects who loved or hated a certain type of music. The results are always the same: The group that disliked the music had more TTS than those who liked it. While "liking" of the music was not protective; "disliking" the music can increase the potential for hearing loss.

Although, to date we have little physiological evidence to explain these findings, the answer may be related to the feedback (or outgoing) neurological pathways that go from the brain, to the outer hair cells in the inner ear (see Chapter 1) as well as the chemistry of the outer hair cells in the inner ear. It is also felt that there may be a change in the circulation in the inner ear on a hormonal basis if music was felt to be beautiful versus terrible. For example, it was found that emotional stress in guinea pigs created increased levels of catecholamines that may reduce the level of available oxygen in the inner ear. Reduced oxygen levels (anoxia) in the inner ear has been suggested as a mechanism for temporary and even permanent hearing loss.

MP-3 players and the 80/90 rule

We have had "portable" music since the development of the transistor radio in the 1950s. In the 1980s we had portable cassette players (e.g. Walkmans), in the 1990s we had portable CD players, and today we have portable MP-3 players such as the ipod. It is the portability of these devices that poses the danger. We can use them while walking by construction sites or on public transit and when this is done, we tend to increase the volume to potentially damaging levels.

What are the damaging levels? It turns out that the 80/90 rule is a good place to start, and this came out of the research of Dr. Brian Fligor. If we listen to music at 80% of the volume setting for 90 minutes a day, this would give us about 50% of our noise "dose" for the day. This is not exact since the earphone used can be the main culprit in how loud the music is, but the 80/90 rule is a good place to start. If your favorite song comes on, turn up the volume and enjoy it; just turn down the volume to 80% or less after. And if you want to listen for more than 90 minutes a day, either turn down the volume further or take the next day off. Like many things in life, moderation and common sense are the key elements.

Smoking and Hearing Loss

Yet, another factor may be that many musicians play in smoky environments and may even smoke themselves. A small, but growing body of research is attempting to answer the exact nature of the interaction between hearing loss and an increased carbon monoxide level such as that found with smoking. However, no definitive study provides conclusive evidence. This is probably related to the fact that those who smoke also have other physiological problems that may alter their susceptibility to hearing loss from music exposure.

There is evidence that cardiovascular function and overall physical fitness can affect the propensity for hearing loss. Scandinavian researchers found shipyard workers who had increases in heart rate and blood pressure when working hard, also had the greatest hearing losses. They studied the degree of TTS initially and after these same subjects completed an eight-month physical training program and found that after the training program there was significantly less TTS. The rationale is that more physically fit people have a better over-all blood supply, including the supply to the inner ear. This increased blood supply implies that those with better cardio-vascular systems (e.g. non-smokers) are less susceptible to hearing loss from loud music or noise. This is also supported with research from the American Medical Association.

However, to muddy up the waters, other researchers found that the effects of smoking and cold temperatures decreased one's susceptibility to hearing loss. They argued that both of these factors cause a peripheral vasoconstriction, thereby making more blood flow available to central locations such as the inner ear. They also found that exercise and smoking in noise decreased one's susceptibility to hearing loss as compared with a nonsmoking, nonexercising group. It was argued that more blood supply was available to the central locations such as the inner ears of the smokers because of the peripheral vasoconstriction of this group. In this same vein, they also found that lower body temperature decreased one's susceptibility to noise exposure.

These findings are not necessarily contradictory. Simply stated, if there is less oxygen and/or more carbon monoxide (from smoking) available to the inner ear, there will be an increased risk to music and noise exposure. In summary, to reduce the propensity for music or noise exposure, if people smoke, then they should make sure their cardio-vascular system is very healthy. Because many smokers do have associated cardiovascular problems and tend to have more overall health problems, they should be counseled to minimize their exposure to damaging music or noise, or at least to take extra precautions to reduce the exposure. So don't smoke and get plenty of exercise.

Chapter 3
Strategies to Reduce Music Exposure

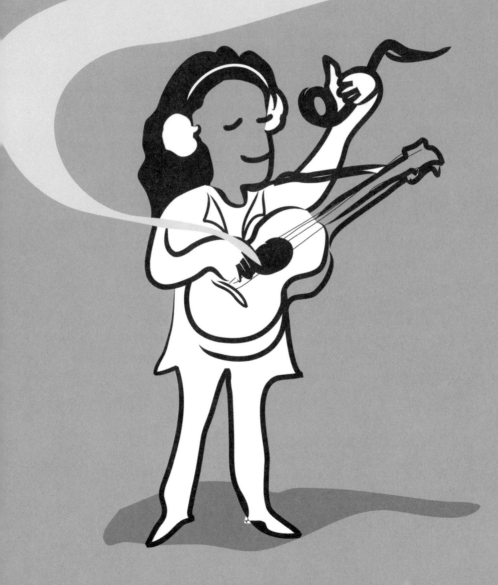

Chapter 3: Strategies to Reduce Music Exposure

Hearing Protection

Many musicians who have tried hearing protection in the past have commented that the sound is hollow and there is "no high-end". There are reasons for these comments and the understanding of the physics behind them have led to much improved and readily acceptable ear plugs. Musicians now have a range of optimal hearing protection at their disposal that will allow optimal hearing with no echoey sensation. The echoey/hollow sensation is related to the occlusion effect and the loss of high-end hearing is related to a fundamental characteristic of sound.

Custom made hearing protection means that the musician goes to an accredited audiology or hearing aid dispensing facility and has custom made ear mold impressions taken. These impressions are sent to earmold laboratories. About a week later, the custom made form of hearing protection is fit. During the fitting session, the hearing health care professional may use a small microphone situated in the ear canal to verify the function of the hearing protection. This can be done while the musician plays their own instrument, as shown in Figure 3-1.

The Occlusion Effect

When we sing, talk, or play a musical instrument, the sound energy of our own voice or instrument not only goes out into the environment, but also goes in to our ear canals. The inner portion of our ear canal is lined with bone (as compared with the outer portion which is cartilage). This bone receives low-frequency sound vibration directly from our jaw and mouth. That is, the boney wall of the ear canal vibrates like a speaker diaphragm and sound is generated in the ear canal. Normally, this sound energy goes out to the environment. However, what happens if we plug up the ear canal with an earplug or our finger? The sound becomes trapped in the ear canal and goes inward through our hearing system—we hear it. This is called the occlusion effect and accounts for the echoey and hollow sound of our voice whenever we plug our ears.

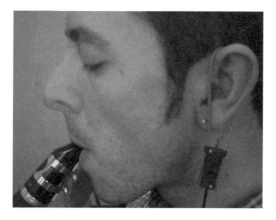

Figure 3-1: Musician being tested with a real-ear measurement system while playing the clarinet. A probe is inserted into the ear canal between the earplug and the ear canal wall while the clarinet is being played.

Understanding the occlusion effect helps in solving it. In order to minimize the effect, a longer earplug is made that extends in to the boney portion of the ear canal. It is like placing one's hand on the cone of a speaker. If you push hard enough, the vibration will not occur—that is, the loudspeaker will not work—with no sound being transduced. If the ear plug is made with a long enough bore extending into the ear canal, it will prevent any vibration from being transduced to the ear. Practically this means that in order to minimize the occlusion effect, one needs to have a custom ear plug that is made with a long ear canal bore. Non-custom, off the shelf products, regardless of how well they fit, will always have some echoey sensation associated with them when worn.

Another solution to minimize the occlusion effect is to create a hole or vent in the ear plug that will "bleed off" the unwanted low-frequency sound energy.

"I have no high-end"

A second complaint about standard hearing protection is that the music sounds muffled with "no high-end". This comment is related to a fundamental characteristic of sound. "High frequencies don't like small spaces". One may characterize higher frequency sounds as being clastrophobic—not liking small spaces. Scientists would say that the acoustic imped-ance of the acoustic inertance is proportional to frequency, but most people agree that scientists can't speak English! They simply mean that low-frequency bass notes go through walls and other obstructions (such as earplugs) without noticing that there is an obstruction. In contrast, the higher frequency treble notes see walls and earplugs as obstructions and tend to reflect, rather than going through. Earplugs then, will al-low the low frequency bass notes to get through but there is "no high-end".

The Occlusion Effect

The occlusion effect is a build-up in the ear canal of low-frequency sound energy from a person's own voice or musical instrument. When an ear is plugged up, a person may report that sound is "hollow" or "echoey". This is not just a perception- this is a real phenomenon that can be measured with scientific instruments.

The "physiology" behind the occlusion effect is that low-frequency sound energy is transduced from the mouth, through the maxilla jaw bone, to the boney portion of the ear canal in the outer ear. The ear canal is about an inch long, with the inner half to a third being made up of bone. The outer portion is made of cartilage.

The boney portion of the ear canal is set in vibration, but normally we are unaware of it because the low-frequency vibration goes out the ear. When the ear canal is plugged up however, this low-frequency sound energy is trapped and continues on through our auditory system- that is, it is heard.

There are two strategies to minimize the occlusion effect. One is to create a custom earplug with a very long ear canal bore portion. The wall of the earplug can sit against the wall of the interior portion of the ear canal which will prevent it from vibrating. No vibration means no build-up of sound pressure and no occlusion effect. It is similar to placing your hand against a loud speaker cone. If one pushes hard enough, no sound will come out. The other strategy is to create a hole in the earplug that will allow the low-frequency sound energy to leak out and thereby reduce the occlusion effect.

The occlusion effect can be measured in two ways. The first is by simply having the musician say the vowels [a] as in 'father' and [i] as in 'beet' with the earplug in place. Normally these vowels are equally loud, but the [i] sound has significantly more low-frequency energy than the [a]. This low-frequency energy can be heard better than that of the [a]. If the [i] is judged to be louder than the [a], there is a significant occlusion effect. If they are roughly the same loudness, then no occlusion effect exists.

Please see Occlusion, pg 37 ☞

☞ *The Occlusion Effect continued*

The other assessment techniques involves the use of a special instrument that is routinely found in most audiology offices. A special microphone called a "probe tube microphone" can be placed in the musicians' ear canal and the extent of the occlusion effect can be measured. In some people, it can be as much as 20 dB! Clearly in this case, the earplug will have to be remade in order to resolve this problem. ❦

Other than the scientists' non-English "acoustic impedance" explanation, another factor is that the ear plug is occupying the outer ear canal. In Chapter 1, it was pointed out that a function of the outer ear was to provide amplification for the higher frequency sounds. If the outer ear canal is plugged up, there is a loss of this natural high-frequency boost, much like a French horn player when they partially plug up the bell with their hand or the trumpet player who uses a mute.

One solution would be to incorporate a specially designed amplifier that puts back the higher frequencies, such that the net effect at the eardrum is a flat or equal attenuation for all of the various frequencies. One such "amplifier ear plug" uses an acoustic network (i.e., no batteries) and is called the ER-15 earplug.

The ER-15 Earplug

In 1988, a manufacturer named Etymotic Research, Inc. (hence the name ER) devised a custom earplug with approximately 15 decibels of attenuation over a wide range of frequencies. The earplug (named the ER-15) has become widely accepted by musicians as well as some industrial workers who work in relatively quiet environments. Figure 3-2 shows the attenuation characteristics of the ER-15 earplug (along with the ER-25 earplug, the vented/tuned earplug, and an industrial-type foam plug for comparison purposes). That is, the ER-15 makes all the sounds of music equally quieter by about 15 dB. Shown another way, Figure 3-3 shows the effect the ER-15 has on the spectrum of a violin while playing the note A (440 Hz) played at a mezzo forte level. Note that the violin spectrum with the ER-15 earplug is essentially parallel to the sound without hearing protection. That is, music sound the same, only quieter.

The design of the ER-15 earplug (and its partner, the ER-25 earplug that provides approximately 25 decibels of uniform attenuation) is remarkably simple. Essentially, a button-sized element (that functions as an acoustic compliance, for those that like physics) is connected to a custom ear mold. The resulting interaction between the button-sized element and the volume of air in the earplug creates a resonance (or amplification) that replaces much of the high-end sound that would be lost with conventional earplugs. The ER- button element is manufactured by Etymotic Research, Inc. but the

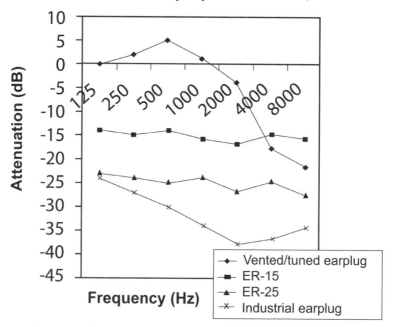

Figure 3-2: Attenuation characteristics of the ER-15 Earplug and that of three other earplugs. Notice how flat the ER-15 and ER-25 responses are.

custom made silicone earplug is made at a local ear mold manufacturing laboratory. Ensuring that the custom made earplug is sufficiently long will minimize the occlusion effect. A schematic and ER-15 is shown in Figure 3-4. In addition to the ER-15 and ER-25, an ER-9 with only about 9 dB of flat attenuation is also available, but these should only be used in rather quiet musical environments.

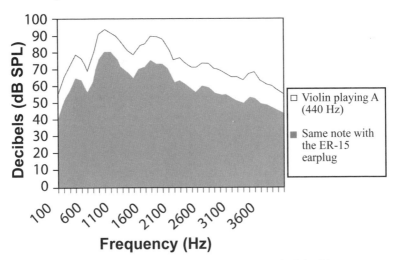

Figure 3-3: Musician playing A(440 Hz) with (black) and without (top) the ER-15 earplug. Note that the 2 curves are parallel, indicating no change in the balance of the music.

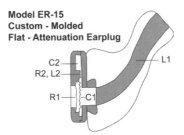

Figure 3-4: The ER-15 earplug uses a combination of cavities, resistances, and volumes to yield a flat (or un-changed) response at the musicians' ear, but with a 15 decibel attenuation. Picture courtesy of Etymotic Research.

A noncustom (and less expensive) product is also available called the ETY (previously called ER-20/HI-FI) earplug and was introduced in 1992. It uses another approach to enhance the higher frequencies and thereby reduce the high-frequency attenuation. Because it is not custom made for an individual's ear, the bore length is necessarily short, and the occlusion effect can be noted. Figure 3-5 shows the ETY earplug.

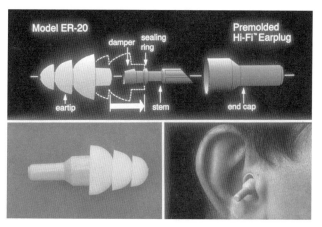

Figure 3-5: The ETY non-custom earplug (previously called the ER-20/HI-FI) is similar to the ER-15, but yields slightly more attenuation (protection) in the higher frequencies. Picture courtesy Elliott Berger, E-A-R, Indianapolis, IN.

The Vented/Tuned Earplug

Another approach to acoustic tuning of hearing protection takes a different slant. Instead of attempting to uniformly attenuate the musical sound, an earplug can be constructed that has minimal acoustic effect in the lower frequencies and a significant high-frequency attenuation. This type of earplug has been in wide use since about 1990. A vented/tuned earplug is a custom earplug with a tuned hole or cavity drilled down the center. The diameter of the hole can be adjusted (tuned) with covers (called select-a-vents [SAV]) that have various sized holes in them. In its most open position, the vented/tuned earplug is acoustically transparent below 2000 Hz, with a significant high-frequency attenuation (up to maximum of 28 dB—with a typical attenuation of 20 dB). Most of the musicians that wear this form of earplug use it in the most open position.

A vented/tuned earplug would allow a musician to hear the lower and mid-frequency sound energy of their own instrument but provide significant attenuation for the high frequency stimuli in the immediate vicinity. Such an earplug is quite useful for woodwinds or larger stringed instruments that have significant high-frequency damaging energy in their environments. For example, a clarinet player will still be able to hear their own music, while the vented/tuned earplug will lessen the intensity of the cymbal crashes from the rear. The attenuation pattern of the vented/tuned earplug is shown in Figure 3-2.

There is a small (4–5 dB) resonance in the 500 Hz region (one octave above middle "C") that is caused by the mass of air in the "vent " or hole, vibrating. This small resonance can be used to improve the monitoring ability of some musicians and some vocalists. It also can be used as part of a program to reduce vocal strain. That is, a small bit of amplification (like the occlusion effect) can improve the awareness of a singer's own voice in a possibly noisy background. Too much of an occlusion effect may be as bad as too little for some musicians.

Modifications of the vented/tuned earplugs are also available that use acoustic resistors in, or in front of, the vent. Ear mold laboratories have different names for these "filtered" vented/tuned earplugs, and the attenuation characteristics will vary depending on the filter used, as well as on the sound bore dimensions.

Table 3-I list the various forms of optimal hearing protection for the various musical instruments. In some cases, more than one type is possible because of the environment that the musician finds themselves in. The input from your local hearing health care professional such as an audiologist will be invaluable. In some cases, more than one type is required for optimal performance if the environments are significantly different. For example, this may be the case for a clarinet player that plays with an orchestra (ER-15) and then plays in a Blue's band (vented/tuned earplug).

Instrument	Auditory Danger	Earplug(s)
Reeded Woodwinds	Brass section to the rear	ER-15 Vented/tuned
Flutes	Flutes (>105 dB)	ER-15 Vented/tuned
Small Strings	Small strings (>110 dB)	ER-15
Large Strings	Brass section to the rear	Vented/tuned
Brass	Brass (>105 dB)	Vented/tuned
Percussion	Percussion (high hats)	ER-25
Vocalists		
Solo	Soprano (>115 dB)	Vented/tuned
Non-solo	Other instruments	ER-15
Amplified Instruments	Speakers/monitors	ER-15

Table 3-I: Summary of various instrument categories, along with the source(s) of potential damage, and the optimal choice of earplug. See text for explanation.

Two Laws of Physics

These two laws are actually related, but manifest themselves differently in enough situations to be treated separately.

(i) A first law is that high frequencies don't like small spaces. A scientist might say that the acoustic impedance is proportional (or increases) with frequency.

Low-frequency sounds, such as the bass notes, have long wavelengths, like the waves in a rolling ocean. As a rule of thumb, in order for something to behave as an obstruction, it has to be at least one half the size of the wavelength. Understandably, a low-frequency sound then needs a very wide obstruction to alter its movement. In contrast, a high frequency sound has a shorter wavelength- that is, it is more frequent.

An obstruction, such as an earplug, may have no effect on a low-frequency sound but would interfere significantly with a higher frequency treble sound. High frequency sounds get caught (i.e., they are interfered with) by holes in acoustic tiles, and even air molecules. Acoustic tiling on ceilings, attenuate or lessen the energy of higher frequency sounds more than bass notes. If one was to measure the intensity of music at the front of an audience, and then measure it again at the back, there would be less relative overall high frequency energy at the back of the hall because of the air molecules interfering with this sound.

(ii) A second law of physics is that higher frequencies are directional.

When sounds emanate from the end of a trumpet bell, the lower frequency bass notes do not "see" the metal wall of the trumpet as anything to be concerned about. Low-frequency bass notes leak out of the trumpet almost everywhere. In contrast, the higher frequency treble notes (have shorter wavelengths) and as such "see" the trumpet wall as a real wall. These sounds are guided out of the trumpet bell in almost a straight line — like a laser beam. Placing the trumpet players on risers will allow the intense beam of sound energy to go over the heads of those other musicians "downwind".

Please see Two Laws of Physics, pg 44 ☞

☞ *Two Laws of Physics continued*

Another example concerns loudspeaker design. Like the trumpet bell, the higher frequencies emanate from a loudspeaker in a much more direct path than the lower frequency bass notes. Elevating the speakers or aiming them at the musician's ear would improve the audibility of these higher frequency sounds, such that, in many cases, the sound engineer or musician would turn down the overall volume. Not only would the music have a flatter response, but it would also be less damaging. ☙

Some Techniques to Reduce Music Exposure

Since different musicians find themselves in differing environments, the strategies to reduce the effects of music exposure may be different. The following is organized around seven "musical instrument" categories, even though there is some overlap. Chapter 4 has some fact sheets summarizing this information, but this will serve as the basis for those summaries: 1) small strings, 2) large strings, 3) brass, 4) woodwinds, 5) percussion, 6) amplified instruments, and 7) vocalists.

1) Small Stringed Instruments

The instruments in this category include the violins and the violas. The ear protection of choice is the ER-15 earplug, as this will provide broadband uniform attenuation that is ideal for these musicians. The violins and violas generate significant low and high-frequency sounds and more importantly, these musicians need to hear the balance between these sounds. Sound levels in excess of 110 dB have been measured even when played at an average, or mezzo forte, loudness.

A very important factor is the positioning of this musician. Violin and viola players should never be placed under an overhang that is within 1 meter of their heads. Such poorly constructed overhangs in "performance pits" are commonplace at many theater, ballet, and opera venues. Space limitations tend to define the size and dimensions of such performance pits. The higher frequency components of these instruments can be absorbed by the underside of the overhang with the result of a loss of hearing of the harmonics. Since the higher frequency harmonic structure is crucial to a perception of proper playing for these instruments, violinists and violists tend to overplay in order to re-establish the correct harmonic balance. Arm and wrist damage can easily result.

Figure 3-6 shows the effect of a poorly constructed overhang on the spectrum or energy of a violin playing the note A (440 Hz), compared with a spectrum of the same note played in "the open." Loss of some high-frequency harmonic energy would not be a problem for some other instrument categories such as clarinet players.

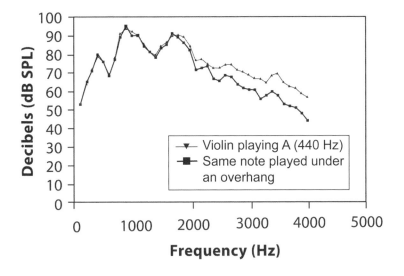

Figure 3-6: A poorly constructed overhang, such as that found in many orchestra pits, can "eat-up" some of the higher frequency sound energy.

Another useful technique for violins and violas is to use a mute while practicing. Such a mute fits over the bridge of the instrument and attenuates or lessens the sound energy by adding an extra mass component to the bridge transduction system. Depending on the style of the practice mute, differing degrees of attenuation may be realized.

2) Large Stringed Instruments

The cello, bass, and harp are the three major instruments in this category. Like all stringed instruments, it is crucial to hear the high-frequency harmonic content; however, because of the larger physical size, most of the important harmonic energy is below 2000 Hz (one octave below the top note on a piano keyboard). Therefore, unlike violin and viola players, placing these musicians under a poorly constructed performance pit overhang will subsequently have little acoustic and ergonomic effect on their playing.

Partly because of the large size of these instruments, the sound levels generated are not excessively great. However, the brass section is typically located to their immediate rear, and it is this source that is the potential threat to hearing loss.

The ear protection of choice is the vented/tuned earplug (see Table 3-I). This earplug serves to allow most of the fundamental and higher frequency harmonic energy of these instruments through to the ear with minimal alteration in the spectrum. However, these earplugs provide significant high-frequency attenuation. The vented/tuned earplug (in its most open condition) therefore can be ideal for the large stringed instruments as it attenuates only the higher frequency sounds of the "noisy" brass section to their rear.

As will be discussed later, belled instruments, such as the trumpet, are highly directional but only for the higher fre-quency sounds. And it is these high frequency treble notes that are the most intense. If the trumpet section is placed on risers, most of the damaging high-frequency energy literally goes over the heads of the musicians "downwind."

Another strategy successfully used by large string instrument players is an acoustic monitoring device. Figure 3-7 shows a schematic of this device that serves to transduce low-frequency energy from the cello or bass directly to the ear. This is analogous to a doctor using a stethoscope.

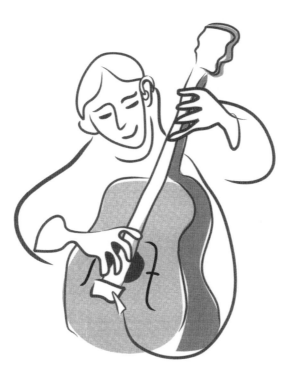

Figure 3-7: An acoustic monitoring device consists of a length of standard hearing aid tubing that joins an earplug (usually a vented/tuned earplug) to a bass instrument. The attachment can be clipped onto the tailpiece, taped to the instrument body, or simply placed in a "f-hole". It is essentially a stethoscope.

Many cello players lean on the pegs of their instrument in order to better hear the low-frequency response that is masked by the rest of the orchestra. This can be inefficient and, in some cases, can lead to neck strain. An acoustic monitor is made up of four feet of standard (#13) hearing aid tubing that is connected to a suction cup at one end and plugs in to the left ear vented/tuned earplug on the other side. The suction cup can be placed on the tail piece of the bass or cello, on the back, or simply sitting in one of the "f-holes". This stethoscope-like device will allow the bass and cello player to hear more of the low-frequency sound from their instrument. Figure 3-8 shows the boost in low-frequency monitoring that can be achieved. This device is very inexpensive and the hearing health care professional can provide such an acoustic monitor to be used with the vented/tuned ear plug or with the ER-15 and a small hole drilled into it.

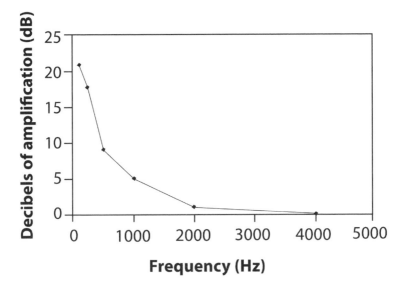

Figure 3-8: Acoustic monitoring device (for cello or acoustic bass) amplifies low-frequency sounds, in order to improve monitoring of one's own instrument.

3) Brass Instruments

Typical instruments of this category are the trumpet, French horn, trombone, and assorted bass instruments such as the tuba and baritone. Two important characteristics are that brass instruments are "directional" for higher frequency energy and that this high-frequency energy is significantly more intense than the lower frequency fundamental energy. The instrument that can generate the most intense music in this category is the trumpet and for this reason it will be used as the example.

The trumpet (and other brass instruments) generates sound that emanates from the end of the bell. Strictly speaking however, this is only true for the higher frequency treble notes. In fact, these treble notes come out of the trumpet bell almost like a laser beam. If measured just below or just above the playing plane of the trumpet, this high-frequency sound energy would not be as intense as if measured directly in front of it.

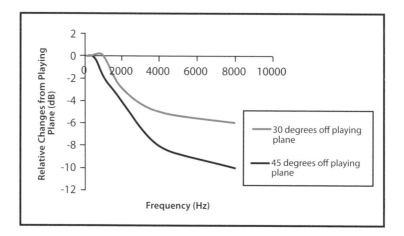

Figure 3-9: Low-frequency bass notes leak out of the trumpet in every direction. However, higher frequency notes emanate in a straight line – almost like a laser beam. This is very similar to what happens in a loudspeaker.

This however, is not true of mid and lower frequency bass notes. These notes leak out of the trumpet and may be just as intense behind the trumpet player as in front of them. Figure 3-9 shows this characteristic of all treble brass instruments. Therefore placing the trumpet players on risers will allow all of the intense high-frequency energy of the trumpet to go over the heads of those other musicians "downwind".

When measured at the position of a cello player's ear in an orchestra where the cellist is "downwind" of the trumpet section, a 5 - 7 dB high-frequency decrease in sound energy was achieved when the trumpet section was placed on risers. This significantly reduced the music exposure for other instruments in the orchestra or band. In addition, when placed on risers, the trumpet players played at a level that was 2 - 4 dB less intense, thereby reducing their own music exposure and embochure stress. Anecdotally, trumpet players report that they tend to be less stressed when they play while on risers. Brass players do not always need hearing protection, but when they do, the ER-15 is the optimal choice because of its flat attenuation response.

Various types of practice mutes are available for brass instruments and these have the general effect of reducing the overall sound levels. Depending on the model used, mutes can be quite frequency-specific, and musicians tend to try several models before they find one that is optimal for their style of playing. Because the more intense sounds of brass instruments are directional (away from the musician), practice mutes are more for the neighbors than for the brass players themselves. Electronic mutes can also be used that not only function as an acoustic attenuator, but also can allow the musician to monitor the music electronically through headphones. Finally, an innovation that has been of great use for French horn players, is the use of a reflective baffle to their rear that is angled back at 45° to the floor. This baffle serves to reflect the higher frequency components of their music to the audience and, incidentally, is a welcome protector for the trumpet players who are unfortunately placed to their rear.

4) Woodwinds

The woodwind category is made up of clarinets, saxophones, flutes, oboes, and bassoons, as the major representatives. These instruments can be played in a wide range of venues, such as in large orchestras or with small jazz and blues bands. In orchestral environments, woodwinds are typically near the front of the orchestra but situated in front of the brass or percussion sections. In jazz and blues environments, they can be in front of speakers or near the drummer.

The ER-15 earplug is recommended for jazz and blues performing venues, and vented/tuned earplugs for the orchestral environments. The rationale for the use of the vented/tuned earplugs in an orchestra is similar to that for the large stringed instruments—namely, to attenuate the high-frequency music energy from other instruments to the rear. The broader band ER-15 earplugs are more appropriate for the more varied music sources in a jazz or blues band.

With woodwind instruments, the sound emanates from the first noncovered finger hole, and as such may be "lost" between the legs and music stands of other musicians. Placing woodwind players in an unobstructed location will allow a direct path for their sound. If the woodwinds' sound is obstructed, overplaying can and does result with the potential of a career-ending injury to the muscle that controls the embouchure. This is also a frequently stated concern of brass musicians.

In the jazz and blues environment, a woodwind player may be situated near a speaker or near the cymbals of the drum kit. In most jazz or blues bands, the drummer hits harder on the ride cymbal (on the dominant side—typically the right side) and the woodwind player should situate himself or herself away from that potential source of music exposure. It is usually the best strategy to situate oneself parallel to a speaker rather than to the front or to the rear of the speaker, as the speaker enclosure wall affords some protection.

5) Percussion Instruments

Whereas there may be some flexibility in the specification of ear protection for other instrument categories, there is very little choice for most percussionists. The ER-25 earplug is the optimal ear protection. Excessive ear protection may result in wrist or arm damage, and too little may result in a progressive music-induced hearing loss. More on this will be discussed near the end of this chapter.

For the full drum kit (with drums and cymbals), hitting the high hat cymbal with a drum stick can be the greatest potential threat to hearing. It is commonplace to find that the hearing in the left ear is worse for a right handed drummer because of the close proximity to the high hat (and the converse for some left handed drummers). The high hat is the main cymbal for rock and roll, with the ride cymbal (on the dominant or, typically, right side) for jazz and blues. The high hat, as the name suggests, is about the diameter of a brimmed hat with two opposing cymbals facing each other. A pedal can be used to move them together or leave them apart. Rock and roll musicians tend to play with the high hats slightly apart, whereas blues and jazz musicians tend to have them apart only about 50% of the time. Figure 3-10 shows two spectra- with the high hats closed and with the high hats open. Note the increased spectral bandwidth and increased intensity when the high hats are left open. Although not shown in these spectra, the duration of the sound of the open high hat will be longer.

The positioning of the high hats is a matter of taste (and music style), and little can be done to convince a drummer to change his or her taste other than by education. However, many drummers are willing to play with a closed position high hat during practice sessions or even to use a muffling practice pad in between the two opposing faces of the high hat cymbal.

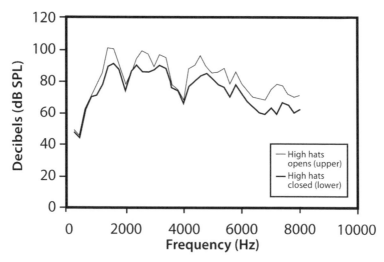

Figure 3-10: The spectra (or display of energy) of high-hat cymbal played open and closed (i.e. together). When played in the closed condition, the overall intensity is less.

Another innovation that derives from the military, has recently been resurrected for drummers (and electric bass players) called seat shakers (or bass shakers). These very low frequency woofer loudspeakers can be hooked in to the amplification system and will generate improved low frequency vibrational feedback. As shown in Figure 3-11, these devices look like large hockey pucks and can be bolted to the underside of a seat or more commonly bolted to a piece of 3/4" plywood that is placed on the floor. During playing, low-frequency vibrational feedback is available to the musician, providing him or her with better monitoring. Drummers using this device, tend not to play as loud with a subsequent reduction in the level of the music. This potentially decreases the risk of arm and wrist injury.

As an alternative to earplugs, personal earphones that replace stage monitors, can also be an option. These earphones (or in-the-ear monitors) can be custom or noncustom. They are essentially in-the-ear hearing aid shells that use a broadband speaker that can handle high-levels with minimal distortion. These are either hard wired to the amplification system or connected to an FM wireless receiver worn on the belt or under the clothes. The music is mixed by the sound engineer and transmitted back to the musician so that there will be optimal monitoring. In the wirelesss situations, the musician is free to move about the stage. Because the effects of the environment are minimized when these earphones are used, the sound levels at the ear are significantly lower than if the musicians were using conventional sound field monitoring

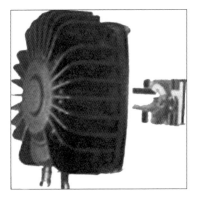

Figure 3-11: Picture of seat (bass) shakers that are low-frequency emphasis speakers designed to improve monitoring of percussion and electric bass. Courtesy of Future Sonics, Inc.

systems such as wedge speakers. Figure 3-12 shows a schematic of a custom earphone system. Several manufacturers market such a system, and while they can be costly, custom earphones are gaining popularity. One such earphone system is shown in Figure 3-13.

A less costly "hard-wired" system can be used by joining a pair of broad band hearing aid receivers to standard (body aid style) earmolds and connecting this to an equalizer/amplifier that can be adjusted for overall gain and frequency response shaping. This has been very useful for percussionists who only need improved monitoring to hear a "click track".

Some recent research has indicated that people still need to be aware to turn down the volume when they wear in-the-ear monitors. It turns out that quieter, less damaging levels, are more acceptable by those who wear the monitors (versus stage monitors) but that unless counselled, people may still wear them at a higher, potentially damaging levels.

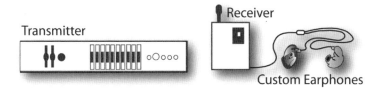

Figure 3-12: Schematic of a custom earphone system for monitoring. The custom earphones can "communicate" with the amplifier either via a wireless (FM) remote as shown above, or can be hand-wired into the system.

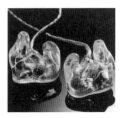

Figure 3-13: A custom earphone is made up of a manufactured earpiece with a cable that can be connected to either a wireless FM system or "hard-wired" to the amplifier directly. Picture courtesy of Ultimate Ears, Inc.

Finally, drummers can use the effect of their stapedial reflex to their advantage. If a loud sound is about to occur, such as by hitting a cymbal, the drummer can begin humming just prior to and through the length of the loud sound. Such humming serves to elicit the stapedial reflex, thus providing some additional temporary ear protection. A discussion of the properties of the stapedial reflex can be found in Chapter 1.

6) Amplified Instruments

Musicians in amplified environments usually have a more flexible work environment than those who work in an orchestra. Rock, blues, and jazz musicians tend to work for themselves and are considered self-employed. Unlike many orchestral musicians, they may have some control over the instrument set-up. Therefore, recommendations of an environmental change for reducing the potential for music exposure are more frequently followed.

These musicians should be either situated away from loud speakers or parallel to the speaker enclosures walls as this will afford some protection. In those cases where loud speakers are oriented towards the musicians in order to obtain "side-wash," the speakers should be elevated. This should be done with caution, as many loud speakers are designed to be placed on the floor. One should check with the manufacturer or retailer before using a speaker in a position that it was not originally intended. Elevating the speakers is done for the same reason as elevating brass players on risers. Like the trumpet, the speaker cone of a loud speaker is highly directional, but only for the higher frequency treble notes. Increasing the height of loud speakers to the level of the performer's ear will improve the monitoring of these higher frequency components, such that the sound engineer will be able to decrease the overall sound level emanating from the loud speaker. The musician will feel that the music is as loud as before, but the overall intensity will be lower, with less potential for hearing damage.

Musicians playing in an amplified environment should be using the ER-15 earplug (except for the drummer who should be using the ER-25). If improved monitoring is required, in-the-ear monitoring (as discussed in the percussion section above) can be very useful. Other than improved monitoring, significant hearing protection can also be achieved with these monitors.

7) Vocalists

By far, the primary concern of vocalists is related to vocal strain. Blues and jazz singers frequently complain of sore throats after long sets, especially in smoky environments. While part of the problem is the air quality, their situation can be improved by the use of an earplug that creates a slight occlusion effect.

Vocalists are divided into two categories: solo and nonsolo. Solo vocalists can be found in classical environments and may be accompanied by relatively quiet instruments. The vented/tuned earplug is the most appropriate protection in this case. These earplugs will provide some high-frequency attenuation, but also will generate a slight increase in the loudness of one's own voice. The vocalist will tend to sing slightly less loud with reduced long-term vocal strain.

Nonsolo vocalists, typically found in pop bands, are susceptible to the same sources of music exposure than their instrumental colleagues. Because of the wide range of music sources on stage, the wide band ER-15 earplug is the form of ear protection of choice. As in the case of the solo performer, a slight degree of occlusion may be useful, and it is therefore recommended that the ER-15 earplugs be made with short canals. Nonsolo vocalists will also gain an improved monitoring (as well as some hearing protection from the various sources of music) by using the custom earphones as shown in Figures 3-12 and 3-13.

Two Hearing/Non-hearing Interactions

The auditory system is certainly not the only potential area of damage for musicians. Entire clinics have been set-up, based on a sports injury model, to provide rehabilitation services and prevention education to musicians. Two forms of musician injury can be related directly to improper auditory or hearing monitoring. These are vocal strain/nodules and wrist/arm injury.

Vocal Strain and Hearing Monitoring

Singers frequently report vocal strain, especially after a long set or if they are required to sing in a smoky environment. Although vocal strain is primarily related to the singing intensity and length of singing time, vocal strain may also be related to monitoring. Monitoring of one's own voice is necessary for the proper speaking and singing intensity.

Improving the monitoring of a singer's voice during a performance by creating a slight occlusion effect has been shown to clinically decrease vocal strain, and in a few cases, has been shown to reduce the severity of vocal nodules. This is a very exciting area of current research and investigations are underway that seek to assess a wide range of voice-related

In-the-ear Monitors

In-the-ear monitors are small custom made loudspeakers that are designed to fit into a musician's ear, much like a small hearing aid. The monitors are fit binaurally (in both ears) and can either be connected directly to the amplifier by a cable (frequently used in this fashion by drummers) or by a wireless FM route.

The advantage of such a monitor is that it replaces the various wedge monitors up on stage as well as the need for "side wash" from speakers aimed sideways up on stage to improve the monitoring of the musicians' own sound. Using in-the-ear monitors means that the environment is controlled and the overall level up on stage is less damaging.

In-the-ear monitors come in two forms – a custom made one and a non-custom one. The non-custom ones uses a foam, "one size fits all" plug that joins it to the ear. An advantage of the non-custom monitor is that the same piece of hardware can be used for different people at different performances- only the replaceable foam plug needs to be changed. A modification of this is to use an inexpensive earmold that is custom made for an individual. The more expensive loudspeaker can connect with this custom made ear earmold which may improve wearing comfort.

In contrast, custom made in-the-ear monitors are made like hearing aids. An earmold impression is taken by a hearing health care professional, such as an audiologist, and sent to a special earmold laboratory. A hard custom made shell is made that fits that individual musician's ear precisely and a miniature loudspeaker is installed in the shell. The in-the ear shell is then connected to a cable that can either be connected directly to the amplification system with an extension cord, or by way of a wireless FM system.

When fitting in-the-ear monitors, there are two issues to consider. One is whether the monitor yields a "flat" response like the ER-series of earplugs and the other is related to the amount of attenuation or protection that the monitor will provide. The in-the-ear monitor will not necessarily have a flat response, but since it is an electrical system, its output can be run through an equalizer to

Please see In-the-ear Monitors, pg 60 ☞

☞ *In-the-ear Monitors continued*

ensure any desired response. As far as the attenuation or protection provided, as a rule of thumb, the softer the material in
contact with the ear, the greater will be the attenuation. A non-
custom monitor that uses a disposable foam plug or one where
an individual musician has had a custom made soft earplug will
provide the greatest attenuation of stage sound. The hard shell
custom in-the-ear monitors will provide less overall protection
from the stage noise than the softer non-custom ones. Using
clinically available probe tube microphones, an audiologist can
measure precisely what the response and the attenuation of an
individual's in-the-ear monitor are, in order to ensure optimal
listening and hearing protection. ❦

measures as a result of improved monitoring caused by a
slight artificial occlusion.

The vented/tuned earplug has been of use in many jazz and
blues venues to reduce vocal strain. Strictly speaking, the
vented/tuned earplug does not significantly increase the occlusion effect. This earplug has a vent-related resonance (see
Figure 3-2) that creates a mild low-frequency amplification.
And it is this slight amplification that serves to improve the
singers' monitoring of their own voice. The ER-15 earplug
can also be modified to create a slight occlusion effect by
intentionally shortening the length of the bore. The short-
ened ER-15 earplug is more appropriate for rock and roll
singers.

Wrist/arm Injury and Hearing Monitoring
Drummers tend to be aware of the potential of music-related
hearing loss. It is commonplace for them to have read in the
popular press that drummers require hearing protection, and
the most available type is the industrial strength earplugs.
Wrist and/or arm strain is the number one reason for drummers
seeking medical help. These two occurrences can be related.

The following scenario is commonly found with drummers: A drummer starts to wear industrial-strength ear protection such as foam plugs, and after about 6 months, arm and/or wrist pain begins.

This problem can be directly related to the wrong ear protection. Industrial-strength foam earplugs attenuate the higher frequency energy to such an extent that there may be a loss of monitoring of the energy from the cymbals and snare drum. Table 3–II shows the intensity of a drummer hitting a practice drum pad (i) with no ear protection, (ii) with the wrong ear protection (foam earplugs), and (iii) with the ER-25 earplugs.

Note that the hitting intensity of the "no ear protection" and the "ER-25 earplug" conditions are similar, whereas that of the "industrial foam earplug" is much greater. In this case, the loss of high-frequency monitoring caused by the foam earplugs caused the drummer to hit the practice pad harder, increasing the potential for arm and/or wrist injury.

Earplug	dBA
Industrial foam earplug	113
ER-25	104
No earplug	103

Table 3-II: Intensity of a drummer hitting a practice drum pad with no hearing protection, with the wrong hearing protection (foam earplugs) and with the ER-25 earplugs.

Hearing Aids and Music

What about those people who are reading this book too late in their musical careers, or are getting up there in age and have a hearing loss? Hearing aids are devices that amplify only certain sounds that are lost. Hearing aids are quite sophisticated in that they make soft sounds louder and almost as importantly, make loud sounds softer. Unfortunately it turns out that hearing aids of 25 years ago were better for music than the more modern digital hearing aids. Hearing aids of the early 1990s were quite capable of re-establishing the dynamics and quality of louder inputs such as music. Modern digital hearing aids are actually better for hearing speech, especially in the presence of background noise, but unfortunately cannot handle louder inputs such as music as well as the older hearing aid technology. Modern digital hearing aids have a great difficulty handling inputs over about 95 decibels and tend to distort.

Engineers are working feverishly to resolve this problem and some improvements have been made. Some ingenious responses have been made, including "auto-ranging" of the hearing aid, to better receive the louder input of music, as well as some other strategies to "fool" the hearing aid into thinking that the input is less intense than it really is. Expect some interesting hearing aid developments for music listening, over the next several years.

If hearing aids are required one should consult their audiologist or other hearing health care professional to determine, not only the best hearing aids, but the best strategies to use them for the listening to, or the playing of music.

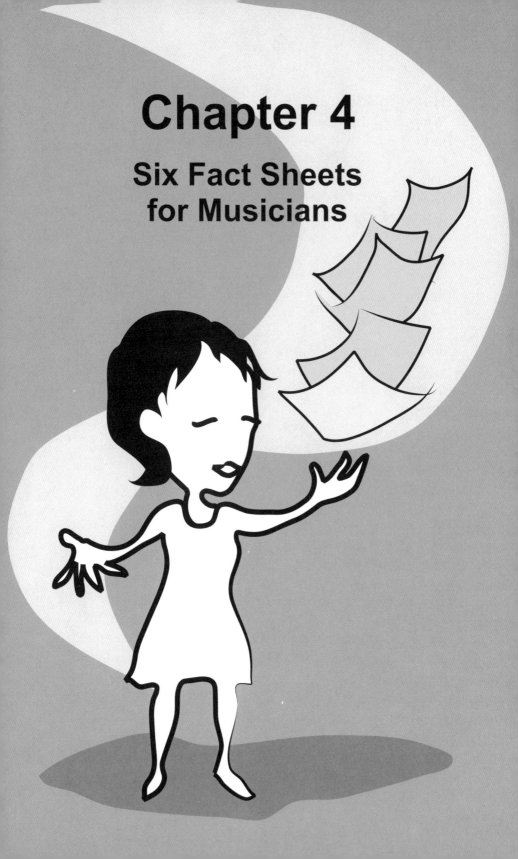

Chapter 4

Six Fact Sheets
for Musicians

Chapter 4: Six Fact Sheets for Musicians

Following are six facts sheets for a number of musical instrument categories that summarize the important strategies to minimize hearing loss from music. There is some overlap, because those musicians that are involved, may have much in common. The science behind these recommendations can be found in Chapter 3.

Each fact sheet can be copied onto a single sheet from your clinic, and be given out to your musician clients.

Guitar and Rock/Blues Vocalists

Guitar players and Rock/Blues vocalists share a similar part of the stage and as such, are similarly exposed to loud music. Some of the strategies to reduce the risk for music related hearing loss, are also similar.

• Ear monitors are small in-the-ear devices that look like hearing aids connected to small wire cables. These can be plugged directly into the amplification system. These not only afford some protection from overly loud music, but allow the guitar players and vocalists to monitor their music better. Frequently, the overall sound levels on stage during rehearsals and performances are quieter while using these monitors. In the case of vocalists, the use of ear monitors will allow them to hear their voice better with an added benefit of reduced vocal strain after a long set. Ear monitors can be designed to either improve monitoring or function as ear protection, or both. Depending on the type of music, one's style, and one's position in the band, a trade-off between these goals may be necessary.

• Loudspeakers generate a wide range of sounds. Like the bell of a trumpet however, not all sounds come directly out of the speaker. Low-frequency bass notes can be just as loud beside the loudspeaker enclosure as directly in front, whereas higher frequency sounds emanate much like a laser beam. Tilting or aiming the loudspeaker up to the musicians' ear will ensure that the music has a "flatter" response. The overall level will tend to be lower on stage because the sound engineer will not need to compensate for a "peaky" response. Some researchers recommend elevating loudspeakers to ear level for much the same reason. Indeed this can be useful, but this will depend on the design of the loudspeaker. Checking with the manufacturer will provide information on whether this is the best choice of orientation for that specific loudspeaker.

• The loudspeakers can also be used as an acoustic shadow to hide in. As stated above, high-frequency sounds tend to emanate from the loudspeakers in almost a straight line. Since these same high-frequency treble notes can also be the most intense, standing beside the loudspeaker enclosure (instead of in front or behind it) may afford some protection.

• The main source of potential damage appears to be from the drummer's high hat cymbal- typically on the left side of the drummer. Moving away from the high hat cymbal as much as is reasonable, or the use of lucite or plexiglas™ baffles between the cymbals and the other musicians may be useful to minimize the potential damage to one's hearing. If baffles are used, it is important to ensure that they do not extend above the level of the drummer's ear, since high-frequency reflections can exacerbate the drummer's hearing problems.

• There are now custom made tuned earplugs that many instrumental musicians and vocalists using called the ER-15 earplugs. These allow all of the music to be attenuated (lessened in energy) equally across the full range of musical sounds. That is, the low-bass notes are treated identically as the mid-range and high-frequency treble notes. The balance of music is therefore not altered. These have been in wide use since the late 1980s.

• The human ear is much like any other body part—too much use and it may be damaged. The ear takes about 16 hours to "reset". After attending a rock concert or a loud session, you may notice reduced hearing and/or tinnitus (ringing) in your ears. And if your hearing was assessed immediately after the concert, one would find a temporary hearing loss. After 16 hours however, your hearing should return to its "baseline" (hopefully normal) level. After a loud session or concert, don't practice for 16-18 hours. Also, its a good excuse not to mow your lawn for a day or two!

Woodwinds and Large Stringed Instruments

Woodwinds such as clarinet, saxophone, oboe, bassoon, and the flute are all found in symphonies and smaller groups. So are the larger stringed instruments such as cello, string bass, and the harp. These instruments generate similar sound levels (albeit at different frequencies), and are subject to similar music exposure from other instruments. Many of these musicians need to sit in front of potentially damaging trumpet and percussion sections.

• Most of these instruments possess significant low-frequency sound energy with very little fundamental and harmonic energy in the higher frequencies. And, these same musicians need to sit "downwind" of the brass section. Most of the damaging energy from the brass section is in the higher frequency ranges, so it would be ideal to have ear protection that lets through the lower frequency sounds, but attenuates (or lessens) the higher frequencies from the other instruments. Indeed such a "vented/tuned ear plug" is useful for these instruments. A tuned cavity is created in the ear plug that allows the musician to hear their own instrument while ensuring that the damaging elements of the trumpet and percussion sections are reduced.

• For those woodwinds (clarinet, saxophone, flute) that also play in jazz and blues bands, a wider form of protection can be useful. These are called the ER-15 earplugs. They allow all of the music to be attenuated (lessened in energy) equally across the full range of musical sounds. That is, the low-bass notes are treated identically to the mid-range and high-frequency treble notes. The balance of music is therefore not altered. These earplugs have been in wide use since the late 1980s.

• Plexiglas™ baffles can be erected between the cymbals and the jazz/blues woodwind players, but should not extend higher than the drummer's ear. Such baffles can attenuate the sound energy of the drums for the other musicians. Ensuring that the baffles do not extend too high, ensures that the drummer is not subject to their own high-frequency reflections, which may increase the potential for future hearing loss.

• In-the-ear monitors are small in-the-ear devices that look like hearing aids connected to small wire cables. They can be connected directly to the amplification system. These not only afford some protection from overly loud music, but allow the woodwind players to monitor their music better. Generally however, these are not necessary unless the music levels are very intense. Frequently, the overall sound levels on stage during rehearsals and performances are quieter while using these ear monitors.

• Acoustic monitors are stethoscope-like devices that can be used by acoustic bass, cello and harp players to allow them to better hear their own instrument. A length of hearing aid tubing plugs into one's custom made earplug on one end and by way of a suction cup or similar attachment, it plugs onto the tail piece, bridge, or body of the bass, cello, or harp. The musician can better monitor their own instrument which has the benefit of not overplaying. Wrist and arm strain is usually reduced with such a set-up.

• The human ear is much like any other body part—too much use and it may be damaged. The ear takes about 16 hours to "reset". After attending a rock concert or a loud session you may notice reduced hearing and/or tinnitus (ringing) in your ears. And if your hearing was assessed immediately after the concert, one would find a temporary hearing loss. After 16 hours however, your hearing should return to its "baseline" (hopefully normal) level. After a loud session or concert, don't practice for 16-18 hours. Also, its a good excuse not to mow your lawn for a day or two!

Bass Players and Drummers

Even though it may be surprising to group bass players and drummers together, because of the similar location in a band, the types of noise exposure can be similar. In some cases, the environmental strategies to minimize the potential from hearing loss, are also similar.

• Humming just prior to, and through a loud sound such as a cymbal crash or rim shot, may afford some hearing protection. There is a small muscle in our middle ears that contracts upon the sensation of loud sounds. This contraction pulls on the bones of the middle ear, thus temporarily making it harder for sound to be transmitted through to one's inner ear. Mother nature designed us with this, so that our own voice would not be perceived as too loud. If one knows about an imminent loud sound such as a cymbal crash, hum just before the crash and sustain the hum through the sound.

• Shakers are small, hockey puck sized speakers that can be wired into the main amplification system. These shakers can be bolted under a drummer's seat, or screwed onto a 1 square foot piece of 3/4" plywood board placed on the floor near the bass player or drummer. The musicians feel they are playing slightly louder than they actually are. The musicians are happy and their ears are happy.

• Plexiglas™ baffles can be erected between the cymbals and the bass players, but should not extend higher than the drummer's ear. Such baffles can attenuate (lessen) the sound energy of the drums for the other musicians. Ensuring that the baffles do not extend too high, ensures that the drummer is not subject to his own high-frequency reflections, which may increase the potential for future hearing loss.

• Ear monitors are small in-the-ear devices that look like hearing aids connected to small wire cables. They can be plugged directly into to the amplification system. These not only afford some protection from overly loud music, but allow the bass players and drummers to monitor their music better. Frequently, the overall sound levels on stage during rehearsals and performances are quieter while using these monitors.

• Acoustic monitors are stethoscope-like devices that can be used by acoustic bass and cello players to allow them to better hear their own instrument. A length of thin hearing aid tubing plugs into one's custom made earplug on one end and by way of a suction cup or similar attachment, it plugs onto the tail piece, bridge, or body of the bass. The bass musician can better monitor their own instrument which has the benefit of not overplaying. Wrist and arm strain is usually reduced with such a set-up.

• Drummers should be using the ER-25 earplugs. Too much ear protection can and does result in arm and wrist strain (due to overplaying) and not enough protection can result in continued hearing loss. The ER-25 (like its more mild form, the ER-15) is a uniform or flat ear protector such that the bass notes, the mid-range notes and the high-frequency notes are all attenuated equally. The balance of music is not altered.

• The human ear is much like any other body part- too much use and it may be damaged. The ear takes about 16 hours to "reset". After attending a rock concert you may notice reduced hearing and/or tinnitus (ringing) in your ears. And if your hearing was assessed immediately after the concert, one would find a temporary hearing loss. After 16 hours however, your hearing should return to its "baseline" (hopefully normal) level. After a loud session or concert, don't practice for 16-18 hours. Also, its a good excuse not to mow your lawn for a day or two!

School Band Teachers

Several inexpensive modifications can be made to school classrooms and portables. Such venues may not be optimal for use as music rooms. These modifications can be accomplished without any special technical knowledge. In addition, other modifications can be made by acoustical engineers. While this second option may be costly, many of the changes made by engineers may yield dramatically improved acoustic environments.

• Trumpets and other treble brass instruments should be placed on risers. Most of the damaging energy of the trumpet is in the higher frequency ranges, and these high-frequency treble notes tend to emanate from the bell of the trumpet like a laser beam. That is, high-frequency damaging sounds will tend to go over the heads of those other musicians downwind. In addition, the trumpet players will not need to play as hard for their sound to be heard clearly. And by the time the trumpet sound reaches the conductor, the levels are not nearly as damaging as for those immediately in front of the trumpets.

• A highly reflective surface, such as a blackboard, behind the teacher/conductor is the worst possible wall covering. High-frequency sounds tend to reflect off such surfaces thereby adding to the overall intensity level in the room. Moveable drapes or thick curtains can be hung over the blackboard (or concrete wall) to absorb these unwanted reflections. They can then be pulled aside when the blackboard is being used.

• Carpeting can be used at the front of the room where the conductor stands. Not only will this absorb some of the un-desirable reflections, but will also allow the music teacher to stand for longer periods of time without backaches.

• 3-D relief art (from the Art Department) would make an excellent wall covering for the side walls of the music room. In this location, the art will not be visually distracting and at the same time absorb many of the undesirable mid- and high-frequency reflections.

• There are now custom made tuned earplugs that many musicians and music teachers are using called the ER-15 earplugs. These allow all of the music to be attenuated (lessened in energy) equally across the full range of musical sounds. That is, the low-bass notes are treated identically as the mid-range and high-frequency treble notes. The balance of music is therefore not altered. These earplugs have been in wide use since the late 1980s.

• The human ear is much like any other body part- too much use and it may be damaged. The ear takes about 16 hours to "reset". After attending a rock concert or a loud session at school you may notice reduced hearing and/or tinnitus (ringing) in your ears. And if your hearing was assessed immediately after the concert, one would find a temporary hearing loss. After 16 hours however, your hearing should return to its "baseline" (hopefully normal) level. After a loud session or concert, don't practice for 16-18 hours. Also, its a good excuse not to mow your lawn for a day or two!

Violins and Violas

Violins and violas can generate sufficiently loud levels of music such that they can cause permanent hearing loss. This is typically worse in the left ear (the ear nearer the instrument). In many cases, the violin or viola player is surrounded by many like instruments, such that the overall level in an orchestra in the violin and viola sections can be quite intense. Unlike most other instrument categories, the ability to hear the higher frequency harmonics is crucial to these musicians. Therefore recommendations are provided to protect hearing and to maintain audibility of the higher frequency harmonics.

• Violins and violas should always be played away from overhangs such as those commonly found in orchestral pits. The roof of such overhangs frequently are treated acoustically in order to minimize reflections. It is not uncommon that the magnitude of the higher frequency harmonic components of these instruments are reduced by this acoustic treatment. Since players of violins and violas need to be aware of this high-frequency energy, the sound is muted. These musicians tend to play harder to compensate for this lost energy with an unnecessary increased sound level and a possible danger to their arms.

• There are any number of acoustic baffles that can be placed on the rear portion of a seat in an orchestra that can serve to reduce the loudness of the instruments to the rear.

Depending on the manufacturer some are opaque and some are transparent. Baffles do work well and serve to attenuate (or lessen) higher frequency sounds more than bass sounds.

However, these seat baffles only work if the baffle is within 7 inches of the musician's ear. If further away, because of reflections off the floor and music stands, the baffles have no significant effect.

• Like other instruments, violin and viola players can use mutes while practising, thus reducing the overall daily exposure to noise/music. These mutes can fit over the bridge and only result in a slight high-frequency loss of musical information.

• There are now custom made tuned earplugs that many violin and viola players are using called the ER-15 earplugs. These allow all of the music to be attenuated (lessened in energy) equally across the full range of musical sounds. That is, the low-bass notes are treated identically as the mid-range and high-frequency treble notes. The balance of music is therefore not altered. These earplugs have been in wide use since the late 1980s.

• The human ear is much like any other body part- too much use and it may be damaged. The ear takes about 16 hours to "reset". After attending a rock concert or a loud musical session you may notice reduced hearing and/or tinnitus (ringing) in your ears. And if your hearing was assessed immediately after such a concert or session, one would find a temporary hearing loss. After 16 hours however, your hearing should return to its "baseline" (hopefully normal) level. After a loud session or concert, don't practice for 16 -18 hours. Also, its a good excuse not to mow your lawn for a day or two!

For those who just like to listen to music: ear plugs, humming and moderation

Hearing loss is a gradual process that may not be noticed for years. And when it does happen, people generally notice that speech is mumbled and unclear. People may report a ringing (or tinnitus) in their ears. By that time, it may be too late. Prevention of hearing loss is where its at! There are many sources of noise in the music industry – explosions, loud cymbal crashes, feedback from speakers, and the routine noise and music of a busy life. Yet, even quiet noises, if one listens to them long enough, can damage one's hearing. A dial tone on a telephone, if listened to long enough, can cause a permanent hearing loss. It's not just rock music – it can be your Walkman, or even a symphony! A permanent hearing loss can be the result of a single loud blast, but more often it's the result of years of exposure to sounds that one would not normally think of as damaging.

• Conventional hearing protection has historically not been well received by those in the performing arts and by music listeners. This form of "foam" plug usually causes the wearer to hear speech as if was muffled and unclear. In addition, frequently one's own voice sounds hollow and echoey. A solution is a tuned earplug called the ER-15 and it treats all sound identically – the low bass notes, the mid-range, and the higher treble notes are all lessened or attenuated by the same 15 decibels. With this earplug, speech is clear and there is significant reduction of the potential for hearing loss from loud sounds. People who wear the ER-15 frequently forget that they are actually wearing ear protection.

• Another strategy is to hum while you work. Humans (and all other mammals) have a small muscle in their middle ears that contract upon loud sounds. From an evolutionary perspective, we have such a muscle so that our own voice would not be too loud for us. When this muscle (called the stapedius muscle) contracts, it pulls on the chain of bones in the ear that conduct sounds, making them less efficient as conductors. Sound from the environment therefore cannot get through to our ears as readily, thus providing us significant protection. If you know that a loud sound or blast is about to occur, start humming before the blast and continue until the blast is finished. Drummers have known this for years without being told.

• Finally, permanent hearing loss starts as a series of temporary hearing losses. When you come out of a rock concert or other loud venue, your hearing may temporarily be decreased. You might noticed this as a muffled feeling and may notice ringing or tinnitus. This temporary hearing loss resolves after about 16-18 hours. Eventually it may become permanent. The strategy would therefore involve moderation. If you see a loud rock group on Friday night, don't mow your lawn on Saturday. Wait until Sunday, or better still get someone else to do it!

Chapter 5
Frequently Asked Questions

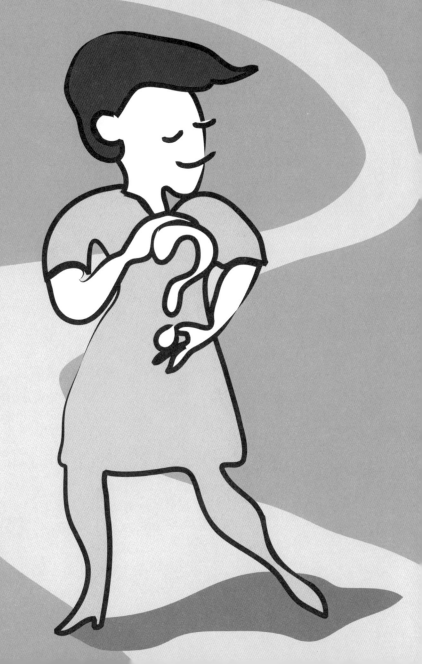

Chapter 5: Twenty-Seven Frequently Asked Questions

1) What happens when we get a music related hearing loss?

Most people reach the ripe old age of 50 without any hearing problems, but others suffer a very slow and gradual hearing loss that may not be noticed for years. Certainly working in a noisy factory is one such cause. And listening to loud music is another. The ear is made up of three parts- the outer ear, the middle ear, and you guessed it, the inner ear. The inner ear is about the size of a small finger nail and contains about 15,500 nerve endings, called hair cells. When some of these hair cells are damaged, you have a permanent hearing loss. Damage to the outer and middle ears is usually temporary and can be treated by a doctor.

2) What are some other causes of permanent hearing loss?

Other than hearing loss associated with aging (called presbycusis), the single greatest cause is working around noise. The ear does not know the difference between loud noise and loud music. To the ear, noise and music are just vibrations in the air. Rarely, a person may suffer a permanent hearing loss from a virus or even a brain tumor. These usually have a sudden onset and may be accompanied by dizziness. Hearing loss from noise or music tends to be gradual in nature with no dizziness. If one experiences dizziness or a sudden hearing loss, one should contact their doctor.

3) Can my hearing loss be treated with medicine or surgery?

Only hearing losses that are from the middle ear (where kids get ear infections) or from the outer ear (such as wax occlusion) can be treated. Rarely can a hearing loss be treated if it is from the inner ear. The inner ear is actually in the brain, so inner ear surgery is brain surgery! Having said all this, researchers are working on a "vaccination" that can be given to reverse inner ear hearing loss.

4) I went to a concert last night and my ears are still ringing. Will this stop?

The ringing is called tinnitus. Actually, tinnitus refers to any noises that are heard in the head, that don't come from the outside. Tinnitus comes in two flavors—objective and subjective. Objective tinnitus is tinnitus that can be heard by other people. This is very rare, and is usually related to blood vessel problems in the ear. Subjective tinnitus is much more common and refers to the type of tinnitus that only the person can hear. But, to answer your question: You are probably suffering from TTS from the concert.

5) Well, ... thank you for that, but what is TTS?

What a good question! TTS stands for Temporary Threshold Shift. This is a fancy way of saying temporary hearing loss. After a loud concert, or a day in the factory, your hearing is temporarily reduced. After about 16 hours to 18 hours, this resolves and your hearing should return to the level it was before (hopefully normal). When the hearing is reduced, there is frequently tinnitus, which is especially noticed in quiet places such as when you are trying to sleep. The tinnitus and hearing loss (sometimes felt as a numbness in your ears) should completely resolve after 16 hours.

6) If my tinnitus goes away after 16 hours, is it safe to go to another concert after?

The short answer is "yes" and "no". It is true that the ear recovers after about 16 hours and can take on new challenges of loud music, but TTS is a warning signal of being exposed to too much music. If you go to a rock concert on Friday night, don't mow your lawn until Sunday (or better yet, get someone else to do it!) However, once you have a music related (or noise related) hearing loss, it is permanent, so do whatever it takes to prevent it. Certainly moderation is one idea. Enjoy that loud song, but when its over, turn down the volume a bit to give your ears a rest.

7) What else can happen as my hearing gets worse?

In some sense, hearing loss is the least of your worries. After all, it is very gradual, and only affects the very high pitched sounds... so you may not notice it for years to come. But, with hearing loss comes two other things that can be very annoying—or if you are a musician, can be career ending. They are pitch perception problems and permanent tinnitus. Pitch perception problems, as the name suggests, means that a person with a significant hearing loss may hear one note as another (and have limited understanding for speech). And can you imagine having a constant hum or whistle in your head day and night? This is what many people report with permanent tinnitus. So, ... prevention of hearing loss is where it's at.

8) So what can be done if I do have tinnitus that won't go away?

Don't panic—this is rather uncommon, but it does occur on occasion. There is almost always a hearing loss associated with the tinnitus. Using a small hearing aid (and there are some that fit invisibly into the ear canal) not only will help you hear better, but will tend to mask or block out the tinnitus in the majority of people. Being overly concerned about it is another problem. The last thing someone should do is become stressed as this may make the tinnitus more noticeable. There are therapy programs that serve to retrain the brain to ignore tinnitus and these can be very successful. Contact your local audiologist or doctor if this becomes a problem.

9) I understand that rock music can be damaging to my hearing, but I can't believe that Mozart or Beethoven can be bad for me.

Believe it or not, but classical music — or specifically playing classical music — can be more damaging than rock music. Research has shown that about 30% of rock musicians have a hearing loss, and about 52% of classical musicians suffer from this problem. The main difference is that classical musicians rehearse, perform, and teach more hours each week than typical rock musicians. And classical musicians tend to be clustered closer together than rock musicians. So even though the peak sound levels in a rock band may be higher than in an orchestra, the total weekly dosage of a classical musician is greater.

10) Are there any other differences between classical musicians and rock musicians besides the obvious?

You mean, beyond the long hair? Although this next issue is highly variable, many classical musicians don't like their music as much as rock musicians do. It is this disliking or hating of the music that is partially responsible for the difference in susceptibility between rock and classical musicians. Research has shown (see Chapter 2) that if you dislike the music, it is actually more damaging than if you like it. Classical or orchestra musicians may play the same piece of music countless times, and become bored with it. In addition, an orchestra musician has their music selected for them by a conductor or artistic director. They may not like the selected pieces. In contrast, a rock musician tends to play their own music—music that they love. This research has been replicated many different ways, always with similar results. So, go ahead and enjoy your music (in moderation).

11) Let me get this straight. If I like my music, it is less damaging to my hearing?

No. It's the other way around. Liking the music will not decrease the potential damage. It's an issue of disliking or hating it that makes music potentially more damaging. We're not sure exactly why that happens, but there are two theories. One is that when you are under stress, certain hormones are released in your inner ear that makes it more susceptible to hearing loss. A second theory is related to the fact that there are a series of feedback loops from the brain back to the inner ear. These feedback signals can change the susceptibility of the inner ear to damage.

12) So what are the factors affecting hearing loss?

The two main factors are how intense the music or noise is, and how long one has been exposed to it. We know from research that prolonged exposure to 85 decibels (dB) or greater, over time will cause a permanent hearing loss. A level of 85 dB is not particularly loud – a dial tone on a telephone is about that! Even though it is not loud, it is intense enough to be damaging. But, it also depends on how long you are exposed to it. Research has found that the maximum exposure each week should be less than 85 dB for 40 hours. This is identical to 88 dB for only 20 hours. That is, for each increase of 3 decibels, you can only be exposed for half as long. Saying it differently, for every 3 decibel increase, your exposure doubles. Other less significant factors are your liking of the music, general health, and hereditary factors.

13) I listen to my MP-3 player at about half volume. Is this level OK?

Well, lets find out. We know that MP-3 players generate about 85 decibels at about 1/3 volume control. Many MP-3 players yield about 95 decibels at half volume. Let's do some math— 85 dB for 40 hours, is the same as 88 dB for 20 hours, which is the same as 91 dB for 10 hours, and this is the same as 94 dB for 5 hours each week. Therefore you can listen to your MP-3 player safely at one half volume for about 5 hours each week. If your favorite song comes on, turn up the volume and enjoy, but be sure to turn it back down after.

14) I have tried earplugs but they sound hollow. Also, I can't really hear the high-end. Are there better earplugs?

Because of the laws of physics, earplugs lessen (attenuate) the sound energy for the higher pitches more than the lower bass notes. Typically earplugs will cause music to sound hollow without much high-end. In the late 1980s, a company named Etymotic Research came out with a "flat" earplug- one that lessens the sound energy for the high pitched notes as much as for the low bass notes. These use a small acoustic amplifier that puts back many of the high pitched sounds. Musicians and music listeners then can hear their music unaffected, except that its at a non-damaging level. These earplugs come in several amounts of protection- 9 decibels of protection (ER-9),15 decibels of protection (ER-15) and 25 decibels of protection (ER-25). Different musicians use different earplug. (See Table 3-I for a listing of which earplug is best for which musical instrument).

15) I'm a drummer and sometimes when I wear earplugs, my wrists hurt. What is happening here?

Wow! Its as if I wrote this question myself! I see this clinically all of the time. Many drummers use industrial strength earplugs, like those used in factories. These earplugs take off a lot of the sound of the high hat cymbal and rim shot of the drum. The drummer needs to hit harder in order to hear properly, with the result of wrist and arm damage. Using proper ear protection will resolve this. Drummers should be using the ER-25 earplug—enough ear protection to prevent further hearing loss, and enough audibility of the music, so that they will not overplay. (For further information, see Chapter 3).

16) I've seen musicians on TV wearing what look like hearing aids connected to small wires. What are these?

These are called in-the-ear monitors, and they are a form of a modified hearing aid. Musicians use them as their own monitoring system instead of the small "wedge" monitors on the floor of the stage. The wires are connected to the sound amplification system either directly or though a wireless transmitter. The musician can then hear their own music as well as that of the other musicians, but at a safe level. When musicians use in-the-ear monitors, the overall sound level on stage is typically much less than if they were using conventional wedge monitors.

17) I play the bass in a band, but can't really hear myself play because the drummer is so loud. Is there anything that I can do?

Unfortunately (for bass players) they usually stand near the drummer. Many bass players (and drummers) use a special type of loudspeaker called a "shaker". These small hockey puck sized devices are designed to enhance the very low pitched bass notes. Shakers are plugged into the main sound amplification system. With this set-up, the bass players and drummers have a better awareness of their own music, and as such, do not have to play as loud. The overall sound level is less, but everyone thinks they are playing louder. The musicians are happy and the music is less damaging.

18) I practice in a small room. What changes can I make to reduce the sound levels... P.S. I don't have much money!

There are some inexpensive changes you can make. Wall coverings and floor coverings are the two easiest things you can do. If there is nothing on the walls, try putting up some heavy drapes. These will absorb many of the undesirable reflections. Also, carpeting will serve the same purpose for those reflections from the floor. A drop ceiling is starting to get a bit costly, but this will also help. Finally, you should be using hearing protection such as the ER-15 or ER-25. These will let you hear your music, but at a safe level.

19) I have seen some clear plastic shields up on stage in front of the drummer. What are these used for and do they work?

These are called baffles and are usually made of Plexi-glas™ or lucite. All baffles, because of the laws of physics, attenuate (or lessen) the intensity of higher pitched sounds more than the lower bass notes. These baffles are designed to lessen the energy for those high pitched high hat cymbals, and rim shot hits that a drummer may make. This protects the other musicians and helps to improve the balance of the music. Note that the low bass thumping sounds from the bass drum are not really affected. The only "trick" with baffles is that they should not extend up above the drummer's ear. The last thing anyone would want is to cause more hearing loss in the drummer by being forced to hear his music, not once, but twice (the initial sound and the reflection off the back of the baffle).

20) I have also seen some baffles hooked onto the back of some seats at the symphony. What are these used for?

These are typically used on the seats of violinists and viola players. In many cases, these musicians need to sit in front of the brass or percussion sections, and they serve to lessen the energy from these louder instruments. The only problem with a seat baffle is that it has to be within 7 inches (18 cm for Canadians, eh?) of the violinist's ear. If it is further away, there is minimal benefit because of the reflections off the floor, ceiling, and music stands.

21) Can I do anything with my loudspeakers to hear better and to protect myself from further hearing loss?

Loudspeakers do not send all sounds out equally. Typically the low pitched bass notes emanate from all parts of the loudspeaker- bass notes are equally loud from the back, front, top and sides. However, the higher pitched notes come out almost like a laser beam- in a straight line. If the loudspeakers can be tilted to aim towards your ears, you will hear a flatter, "more true" sound. And, more importantly, if the loudspeaker is aimed at your ears, the overall volume control level will be lower. In this way, even though the music will sound as loud, it will be less intense. That means it will be less damaging. Intensity is what causes hearing loss, whereas loudness is simply your impression of the sound. Some researchers suggest elevating the loudspeakers, and this can be useful, but be careful. Some loudspeakers are designed to be left on the floor. Check with the manufacturer or retailer before you elevate loud speakers to see if this would be a problem.

22) When I go to a concert in a large venue, the band is set back from the edge of the stage. Is this to protect them from the fans?

How observant you are! It may be to protect them, but there is an acoustic reason as well. The lip of the stage in front of the band or orchestra acts as an acoustic mirror. That is, the higher pitched sounds of the band not only come off the stage to the audience but also reflect off the lip of the stage, thereby enhancing the higher pitched sounds. The band members don't have to play as loud up on stage in order for the people in the audience to hear it better. Not only are the musicians performing at a safer level, but the potential for arm and wrist injuries are lessened.

23) My friend is a drummer and whenever he practices, he hums and grunts. Is he weird or is he doing this for a reason?

He isn't weird (... well, he might be...) but many percussionists hum and grunt. There is a small muscle in the middle ear that mother nature gave us so that our own voice would not be too loud to ourselves (called the stapedial muscle). It has been shown that if one hums or grunts just prior to a loud sound and continues that hum through the sound, this muscle in the ear continues to contract, providing an attenuation (or lessening) of the sound energy. So your friend is actually protecting his hearing. Some of the function of the stapedial muscle is discussed in Chapters 1 and 2.

24) I teach music in a high school and the room is awful. Is there anything I can do to improve it? ... P.S. I don't have much money!

Actually there are several things you can do that are easy to accomplish and inexpensive. Incidentally, there is a fact sheet on this topic entitled "School Band Teachers" (see Chapter 4). You can place the trumpet players on risers as this will allow the higher pitched harmonics of the trumpet to literally go over the heads of the other musicians "downwind". You can put up some drapes over the blackboard behind you while you are playing in order to dampen the unwanted reflections. These drapes can be pulled aside when you want to use the blackboard. Finally, get the Art Department to make some 3-D relief art that can be placed on the side walls. This will also help to lessen the unwanted reflections. High school band teachers, because of the number of hours each week that they must be in a band room should consider the ER-15 earplugs.

Teachers are at risk of hearing loss and have successfully won cases with the Worker's Compensation Board or other regulatory government agencies, in the past.

25) Do you have any specific information or suggestions for bagpipers?

Bagpipes are a fascinating instrument – the only "modern" instrument with no volume control! The output of bagpipes has been measured at 108 dB, and combine that with the drum corps to their rear and you can have a real problem. The hearing protection of choice is the ER-15 earplug if the piper is solo and the ER-25 earplug if drums are around. Of course, the same precautions/moderation should be taken as other woodwinds. You can check out the "Woodwind" fact sheet in Chapter 4 for more information.

26) What earplugs do you suggest for musicians?

There are three major types of ear plugs for musicians – the ER-15, the ER-25, and vented/tuned ear plugs. The ER-25 is generally only recommended for drummers. The ER-15 is the ear plug of choice for most other rock and blues instruments, as well as most classical instruments. The vented/tuned ear plugs are useful for those instruments that either do not have much treble sound energy (such as the acoustic bass and cello), or for those instruments that are not particularly damaging (such as the clarinet), but have to play near other noisy instruments, such as the drums.

27) Where can I get musician ear plugs?

Musician ear plugs, like the ER-15, can be obtained from anyone that makes hearing aids. I would contact an audiologist and they can either make the ear plugs for you, or send you to someone who specializes in musicians. Remember however, that while ear plugs are very important, they are only one of the many things that can be done to reduce music exposure. Environmental strategies (many of which are inexpensive) can be very useful.